ETHICAL
CHOICES

ETHICAL CHOICES

CASE STUDIES FOR MEDICAL PRACTICE

SECOND EDITION

EDITED BY LOIS SNYDER

AMERICAN COLLEGE OF PHYSICIANS

PHILADELPHIA

Manager, Book Publishing: Diane McCabe
Production Supervisor: Allan S. Kleinberg
Senior Production Editor: Karen C. Nolan
Interior and Cover Design: Lorraine Lostracco
Composition: Wendy Smith

Manufactured in the United States of America
Printing/binding by Versa Press

Library of Congress Cataloging-in-Publication Data

Ethical choices : case studies for medical practice / Lois Snyder, editor.—2nd ed.
    p. cm.
    Includes bibliographical references and index.
    ISBN 1-930513-57-7
    1. Medical ethics—Case studies. I. Snyder, Lois, 1961-
    R724.E784 2005
    174'.2—dc22   2004059497

A similar version of each of these case studies has been previously published in ACP Observer.

05 06 07 08 09 / 10 9 8 7 6 5 4 3 2 1

To my daughter,
Hannah

CONTRIBUTORS

Robert A. Aronowitz, MD
Associate Professor
Department of History and Sociology
　of Science
University of Pennsylvania
Philadelphia, Pennsylvania

Anne-Marie J. Audet, MD, FACP
Assistant Vice President
The Commonwealth Fund
New York, New York

Troyen A. Brennan, MD, JD, MPH, FACP
Professor of Medicine
Harvard Medical School
Professor of Law and Public Health
Harvard School of Public Health
Boston, Massachusetts

Richard J. Carroll, MD, SCM, FACC
Executive Medical Director for Quality
Adventist Health System
Hinsdale, Illinois

David Casarett, MD, MA
Assistant Professor of Medicine
Division of Geriatric Medicine
Department of Medicine
University of Pennsylvania
Philadelphia, Pennsylvania

Cynthia Clagett, MD
Honolulu, Hawaii

Errol D. Crook, MD
Assistant Professor of Medicine
Division of Nephrology
University of Mississippi Medical
　Center
Jackson, Mississippi

Frank F. Davidoff, MD, MACP
Editor Emeritus
Annals of Internal Medicine
Philadelphia, Pennsylvania

Kathleen L. Egan, PhD
Director, Geriatrics Education Center
Division of Geriatric Medicine
University of Pennsylvania
Philadelphia, Pennsylvania

Vincent E. Herrin, MD, LCDR, MC, USN
Assistant Professor
Department of Medicine
Hematology/Oncology
National Naval Medical Center
Bethesda, Maryland

Alan L. Hillman, MD, MBA, FACP
Director, Center for Health Policy
Leonard Davis Institute of Health
　Economics
Associate Professor of Medicine
　and Health Care Management
School of Medicine and the Wharton
　School
University of Pennsylvania
Philadelphia, Pennsylvania

Jason Karlawish, MD
Assistant Professor of Medicine
Division of Geriatrics
Department of Medicine
Fellow, Center for Bioethics
University of Pennsylvania
Philadelphia, Pennsylvania

Risa Lavizzo-Mourey, MD, MBA, MACP
President and CEO
The Robert Wood Johnson Foundation
Princeton, New Jersey

Bernard Lo, MD, FACP
Professor of Medicine
Director, Program in Medical Ethics
Division of General Internal Medicine
UCSF Department of Medicine
San Francisco, California

Joanne Lynn, MD
Director, Washington Home Center for
  Palliative Care Studies
Senior Researcher, RAND Corporation
President, Americans for Better Care of
  the Dying
Washington, DC

Barbara Messinger-Rapport, MD, PhD, FACP
Department of General Internal
  Medicine
Cleveland Clinic Foundation
Cleveland, Ohio

Karine Morin, LLM
Director, Ethics Policy
Secretary, Council on Ethical and Judicial
  Affairs
American Medical Association
Chicago, Illinois

Peter Poon, JD, MA
Health Science Specialist
Office of Research Compliance &
  Assurance
Department of Veterans Affairs
Washington, DC

Gail Povar, MD, FACP
Clinical Professor of Medicine and
  Health Sciences
George Washington University School of
  Medicine and Health Sciences
Washington, DC

Miriam Shuchman, MD
Clinical Assistant Professor
University at Buffalo School of Medicine
Department of Psychiatry and Center for
  Clinical Ethics and Humanities in
  Health Care
Buffalo, New York

Lois Snyder, JD
Director, Center for Ethics and
  Professionalism
American College of Physicians
Adjunct Assistant Professor
University of Pennsylvania Center for
  Bioethics
Philadelphia, Pennsylvania

Daniel P. Sulmasy, OFM, MD, PhD, FACP
Sisters of Charity Chair in Ethics
John J. Conley Department of Ethics
St. Vincent's Hospital and Medical
  Center
New York, New York

Kim M. Thorburn, MD, MPH
Health Officer
Spokane Regional Health District
Spokane, Washington

Susan W. Tolle, MD, FACP
Director, Center for Ethics in Health
    Care
Oregon Health Sciences University
Portland, Oregon

James A. Tulsky, MD, FACP
Director, Program on the Medical
    Encounter and Palliative Care
Associate Professor of Medicine
Duke University and VA Medical
    Centers
Durham, North Carolina

Peter A. Ubel, MD
Associate Professor
Internal Medicine Department
Director, Program for Improving
    Health Care Decisions
University of Michigan Medical School
Ann Arbor, Michigan

Janet Weiner, MPH
Associate Director for Health Policy
Leonard Davis Institute of Health
    Economics
University of Pennsylvania
Philadelphia, Pennsylvania

ACKNOWLEDGMENTS

Thanks are owed to the contributors to this collection of case studies, and to the individuals who served and serve on the American College of Physicians Ethics and Human Rights Committee who helped to guide the development of the series. Committee chairs have included Edwin P. Maynard, MD, MACP, Christine K. Cassel, MD, MACP, Lloyd W. Kitchens, Jr., MD, FACP, Risa Lavizzo-Mourey, MD, MBA, MACP, and William E. Golden, MD, FACP, the current chair. Committee members have included Elias Abrutyn, MD, MACP, Troyen A. Brennan, MD, JD, MPH, FACP, Richard J. Carroll, MD, SCM, FACC, Cynthia L. Clagett, MD, Karen E. Coblens, MD, Errol D. Crook, MD, Harmon H. Davis, II, MD, FACP, Susan Dorr Goold, MD, Lee J. Dunn Jr., Esq., Kenneth V. Eden, MD, FACP, Carola Eisenberg, MD, Arthur W. Feinberg, MD, MACP, David A. Fleming, MD, FACP, Susan E. Glennon, MD, Alan L. Gordon, MD, MACP, Vincent E. Herrin, MD, LCDR, MC, USN, Virginia L. Hood, MD, MPH, FACP, Jay A. Jacobson, MD, FACP, Stephen R. Jones, MD, FACP, Allen S. Keller, MD, Bernard Lo, MD, FACP, Joanne Lynn, MD, Steven H. Miles, MD, FACP, John A. Mitas II, MD, FACP, Steven Z. Pantilat, MD, FACP, David W. Potts, MD, FACP, Gail Povar, MD, FACP, William A. Reynolds, MD, MACP, Bernard M. Rosof, MD, MACP, David L. Schiedermayer, MD, FACP, Daniel P. Sulmasy, OFM, MD, PhD, FACP, Siang Y. Tan, MD, FACP, Gerald E. Thomson, MD, MACP, Susan W. Tolle, MD, FACP, and James A. Tulsky, MD, FACP.

Gratitude is also expressed to the staff of *ACP Observer*—where similar versions of these case studies were originally published—and to its Executive Editors during that time, Edward Doyle and Paula S. Katz. I am also indebted to Laura Gregory for assistance with preparation of the manuscript and to Emily Mok for assistance in preparing the annotated bibliographies for this second edition.

And, for always, my love and thanks to Hannah, my daughter, who makes it all clear.

Lois Snyder, JD
June 2004

TABLE OF CONTENTS

PREFACE

The more things change, the more they stay the same. Sort of. The first edition of *Ethical Choices: Case Studies for Medical Practice* was published in 1996. This second edition includes new case studies on topics that have long been the subject of medical ethics debates such as futility, organ donation/procurement, and physician treatment of relatives. Others, however, offer twists on classic subjects. For example, research ethics issues take on a new light when the investigator is the treating physician and the setting is the physician's office. Also addressed are the issues that have emerged from new debates, born of changes in the health care system and in patient expectations about care: complementary and alternative medicine, direct-to-consumer advertising of prescription medications, and technological advances such as genetic testing. Additionally, the number of aging Americans is increasing, as the Baby Boomers (perhaps the world's most demanding and rights-conscious generation ever) bring new meaning to the phrase "coming of age." This will add new wrinkles to old issues, not to mention bad puns, and new urgency to topics such as the older impaired driver.

The case studies in this collection were developed from 1990 to 2003 under the auspices of the Ethics and Human Rights Committee of the American College of Physicians. The commentaries accompanying each case history expand on principles contained in College policy, mostly as found in the fourth edition of the ACP Ethics Manual. (The fifth edition is scheduled for publication in 2005.)

Topic selection usually centers on common ethical problems in medical practice. This volume, however, is by no means comprehensive. The case study series is ongoing, so reader comments and topic ideas are encouraged.

For this new edition, an annotated bibliography has been added to each case study. The purpose of the bibliographies is to guide the reader to the latest and best sources of information. Nearly all of the articles cited can be found in readily available medical journals.

I originally conceived the case study series with three goals in mind: to make principles more relevant to the daily practice of medicine by exploring their application in specific common situations; to ask the reader to think about issues that are important but, being largely the stuff of everyday medical encounters, often are not glamorous; and to demonstrate medical ethics in action while considering the real motivations behind behavior.

Hopefully, these goals have been met on some level, for practitioners, patients, students, and policy makers.

Lois Snyder, JD

FOREWORD
TO THE FIRST EDITION

In recent years, debate has begun in the field of medical ethics about frameworks for the discussion and analysis of medical ethics problems. Rather than starting exclusively from assumptions about ethics drawn from historical values of the profession, such as the Hippocratic oath, or universal rules such as "Always prolong life" or "Never tell a lie," philosophers have articulated ways in which different value paradigms may result in different approaches to the resolution of specific ethical dilemmas. For example, traditional frameworks included various "rule-based ethics," while others claimed that "situation ethics" was more relevant to real-life situations. Situation ethics allows specific circumstances to influence the rule; for instance, a patient suffering from severe depression might not be given full information about a new diagnosis of cancer until the depression had been treated. Newer debates have added feminist ethics, historical or social contexts for ethics, and others as well.

This book recognizes that for physicians, a case-based approach to problem solving is a traditional and time-proven way of approaching problems in medicine. Those of us who have taught ethics on the wards, at the bedside, in the outpatient setting, and in the nursing home know that using individual cases in all their complexity has been the most effective way to teach medical ethics to medical students and residents. We believe that the case-based approach is also the key to understanding medical ethics but that the clinical case for ethics requires a fuller "story" for the values at stake to be understood.

Kathryn Hunter describes the physician's way of thinking in her book *Doctors' Stories,* published in 1994. In it, she recounts the experience of witnessing numerous medical rounds in which cases were presented by trainees. A Socratic form of analysis was used by attending physicians to help elicit an approach to discovering the patient's diagnosis and determining the best approach to management. Hunter compares this process in medicine to that of Sherlock Holmes in his legendary pursuit of the solutions to mysteries. What is fascinating about the Sherlock Holmes metaphor is the way in which Holmes pieced together disparate kinds of information in order to create a story and that the story, when it becomes lucid and credible, becomes a compelling explanation for a series of otherwise mysterious actions and occurrences. It is the stories, thus, that tell us most about the complexity of the interaction of medical practice and conflicts or moral dilemmas. In *Ethical Choices* the case study as "story" is used to best advantage.

Stories are the basis for learning about practical ethical problems in medicine. They provide the foundation upon which abstract analysis can and should be grounded. The various commentaries accompanying each case in this volume should help the reader to better understand the substantive issues raised by specific cases and how to formulate a sustained rationale for an ethical argument. While in the world of medical practice it is the outcome of the story that matters, in the world of medical ethics it is the assessment of action, the evaluation of conduct, and the rationale supporting moral evaluation that matter.

A key reason ethical issues in health care are so riveting and so compelling is that they illustrate how real people in real-world situations make hard choices about important matters. *Ethical Choices* takes full advantage of this richness in the clinical setting.

An especially troubling flaw of other writings in medical ethics is their narrow focus on dilemmas occurring in the practice of highly specialized forms of medicine, which are often at the frontiers of innovation and technology. For every article written about the ethics of telling patients the truth about their diagnoses, there are at least as many, and probably more, about the ethics of using baboon hearts as bridges to transplants that use hearts obtained from human cadaver donors. *Ethical Choices* however, provides a broader perspective to the narrow focus of much of bioethical writing by taking clinical practice and clinical experience seriously. The office, the nursing home, the ambulatory care clinic, and the Urgiclinic are as likely to be locales in which ethical issues arise as are the intensive care unit or the transplant suite. Additionally, patients need not be on the verge of death or critical illness to confound the doctor with difficult and challenging ethical puzzles.

Ethical Choices also points the reader toward the need to understand how good ethics and good medical practice go hand in hand. All too often ethics is seen as somehow at odds with, or as an obstacle to, what the doctor's training and judgment require. It is true that ethical concerns are raised only when suggested courses of conduct deviate from the norm or when a breach in standard practice is proposed. However, it is not true that ethics is only of interest when something outside the mainstream of medical practice is contemplated. As many of the cases in this book make very clear, the clinical practice of medicine is never very far removed from its normative moral base. Doing good and avoiding harm are such foundational principles of medicine that the successful practice of medicine requires a physician who is reflective about applying knowledge and skills to specific instances of disease, illness, anxiety, and disability, be they ordinary or extraordinary cases.

Experienced physicians in practice will find this book useful because it moves from real experience to theoretical analysis, rather than beginning with theory. Students will also find *Ethical Choices* useful because its content and format is consistent with the way they learn in medicine. It ranges from dramatic life-and-death decision making to moral problems that arise in the interactions of everyday practice life, such as economic conflicts and relationships with peers.

None of the problems discussed are simple or can be adequately examined by a general appeal to "rules." Nevertheless, guidelines and principles of medical practice as articulated by the American College of Physicians in its widely cited Ethics Manual are the basis for the resolution of the cases to follow. Together, *Ethical Choices* and the Ethics Manual provide a firm foundation for medical ethics in the practice of modern medicine.

Ethical Choices belongs on every practitioner's shelf. It is an amazing cornucopia of clinical conundrums and everyday dilemmas thoughtfully presented and carefully scrutinized. Those who worry that too much of bioethics is done from the perspective of the armchair will find no reason for concern in these pages. The case material is timely and detailed, and the commentaries and advice are practical and down to earth. Health care professionals and others looking for realistic advice about the daily moral life of medical practice will find helpful insight in the cases that Lois Snyder and her colleagues have written.

Christine K. Cassel, MD, MACP
President, American Board of Internal Medicine

Arthur L. Caplan, PhD
Chair, Department of Medical Ethics
Director, Center for Bioethics
University of Pennsylvania

Introduction to Medical Ethics

Lois Snyder

Medical ethics has come of age. It is no longer the exclusive province of philosophers, theologians, theoreticians, or medical and legal academics. From AIDS dilemmas and doctor-patient sexual relationships, to physician-assisted suicide and the withholding or withdrawal of life support, medical ethics is very much on the minds of patients, practitioners, policy makers, and the media.

Medical ethicists have joined the ranks of talk show guests and news article commentators. This celebrity is good. Talk is good. But in the realm of ethics, talk is ultimately most important to the extent that it leads to action—appropriate action.

This collection of case studies is directed toward action: What should the physician do when facing an ethical dilemma? Principles are pondered, abstractions are analyzed, theory is thought through, arguments are articulated—good discussion is critical to practicing good medical ethics. But in the end, in addition to showing *how* to make ethical decisions in the practice of medicine, guidance as to *what* constitutes the best ethical course in particular circumstances is provided in most instances.

Patients will find the issues contemplated in these cases pertinent to their health, welfare, and rights, and physicians and physicians-to-be will find them relevant to everyday practice. Patients and their physicians, and the relationships they develop or hope to develop, are under increasing pressure from changes in health care financing and delivery, technological advancement, the law, and demographic shifts. Although gene therapy, animal-to-human organ transplantation, and other highly controversial issues often shine in the bioethics limelight, more routine issues like the financial incentives inherent in fee-for-service medicine versus managed care, the impaired doctor, and patient preferences for referrals are often more relevant for practitioners and their patients. The cases included here examine frequent bedside clinical issues and common issues of professional ethics in medicine.

What is *medical ethics?* First, what is *ethics?* Webster's dictionary defines ethics as a theory or system of moral values. I would define ethics as what we should do and why. Ethics is also about the traits and qualities people ought to have or strive to have: the old-fashioned but never out-of-fashion notion of virtue, of good being done by good people. It is not merely about what you feel in your gut is right or wrong, although this is often a good starting point. It is not just about philosophical and other principles, ideals, and rigorous arguments, although these are a large part of practicing ethics. It is not only about what the law, a set of socially determined moral minimums, or tradition, require. It is about all of these things. But it is never simply a matter of consensus. You cannot just vote to determine what is ethical, although if families, schools, the law, politics, the professions, religion, and culture are doing their jobs, you may happen upon an ethically valid vote.

Bioethics encompasses ethical dilemmas in health care, medicine, and the life sciences, combining both theory and practice. Bioethics as a field is still relatively young, with its formal beginnings in the 1960s and 1970s. Responses to research scandals of the day, such as the Tuskegee syphilis "study," plus a series of reports issued by the President's Commission for the study of Ethical Problems in Medicine and Biomedical and Behavioral Research on diverse topics such as informed consent, access to health care, genetic screening, and the refusal of life-sustaining treatment, helped to lay a foundation for the field. Those issues are still very much alive, along with others raised by scientific advances, changing modes of health care delivery, more knowledgeable and demanding patient-consumers, and developments in the law, politics, economics, and culture.

For most patients most of the time, bioethics means medical ethics: the care that they receive from their doctors, the science and art of science that directly touches their lives. If ethics is the soul of medicine, and I believe that it is, then the patient-physician relationship is surely the soul of medical ethics.

Two key principles guide all medical ethics inquiries, especially those that involve the interactions between physician and patient: beneficence, the duty to do good and to act in the best interest of others, and non-maleficence, the duty to do no harm. More recently, two additional principles have been added to the bioethical equation: respect for autonomy, the individual's right of bodily self-determination, and justice, with a focus on considerations of fair treatment and distribution of resources.

A listing of principles, alone, however, will not take you very far down the road of thoughtful ethical inquiry. For example, many commentators invoke patient autonomy as the key, or sometimes the only, aspect of their argument supporting euthanasia or physician-assisted suicide. But they fail to consider the ethical, moral, and social heart of the matter they raise: Autonomy for what? What are the purposes and consequences of such self-determination? Euthanasia and physician-assisted suicide are complex issues. There are good arguments to make in response to the above questions, but arguments that rely on mantras are not very helpful.

When all is said, however, something must be done. Individuals must be aware of ethical issues in health care, confront them, reason through them, and then act. Good bioethics provides good reasons for action. A few examples from the cases:

- When a physician makes a mistake and does not follow up on a test result as he should, there are principles at stake and, more importantly to the patient, there are consequences. The physician must act as an ethical matter, and he must act as a practical matter, lest he be acted upon (by, for example, a malpractice attorney or a disciplinary body).
- When a potential new Medicaid patient or a patient with HIV shows up at the doctor's door, the doctor must decide whether to accept the person as a patient.
- When a patient wants care that the physician thinks is not medically necessary or appropriate, the doctor must decide what to do and say, and the patient must decide how to respond.

Much of what many physicians already do in clinical encounters without extensive reflection is based on what I think is an intuitive sense about what is ethical and appropriate in a given situation: their actions are part of a mindset and worldview born of the culture of medicine and the character and values of the men and women who choose medicine as their profession and their life. With millions of clinical encounters a day, ethical problems are not derailing patient care.

However, there is still plenty of room for refinement and improvement of patient care. The culture of medicine has had its downside. A notable example is the profession's collective behavior in the bad old days before the firm establishment of full disclosure, informed consent, and shared patient-physician decision-making. For some patients, a decision about decision-making means requesting not to be told all the details and granting authority to the doctor to climb the decision tree alone, or to take it up with family members. And there are, of course, appropriate limits to the care a patient may demand, although defining those limits is thought by some to be among the hardest questions in bioethics today.

Physician practice instincts infuse medical ethics deliberations with judgment, passion, compassion, hope, bias, and more: these are, after all, what cause people to act. We need to consider the very real aspects of what people do and why in our consideration of ethical problems. Analysis of motives and resultant actions provides another reason for the case study format used here. Just as most law arises in the context of specific cases with specific fact patterns, medical cases can provide a foundation for practical medical ethics. Additionally, a dry analysis of principles devoid of meaningful context probably will not motivate a busy practitioner or stressed student to finish reading the page on which it is written, let alone incorporate ethics analysis into the way he or she acts or feels. Case studies as an ethics-education tool, especially cases about common problems, can potentially help make more behavior more right, more deliberate and, to the proper extent, more rational.

But not too rational. Principles and rules, whether about substance or procedure, are not moral actors. We are.

Part I

The Patient and the Physician: The Clinical Encounter

The patient-physician relationship defines *how* patients seek care and comfort and is a large element of *why* most physicians practice medicine. The relationship entails rights and responsibilities, ethical and legal, for both the physician and the patient, an obvious but central guiding fact. Care is a joint endeavor.

Many types of clinical encounters could serve as the basis for thought-provoking case studies. Part I highlights several important issues including futility, genetic testing, alternative therapies, physician-assisted suicide, and organ procurement.

1

Deciding How Much Care Is Too Much

Commentary by James A. Tulsky, MD, and Lois Snyder, JD
Case History by James A. Tulsky, MD

Case History

Sandra Jones, an 83-year-old woman with Alzheimer's-type dementia, severe osteoarthritis, and type II diabetes mellitus, has been a resident of the Greenview Nursing Home for 5 years. For many years, Mrs. Jones lived with her daughter and son-in-law, but as her mobility decreased caring for her became exceedingly difficult. Four years ago, Mrs. Jones' children reluctantly admitted her to the nursing home.

One year after being admitted, Mrs. Jones developed end-stage renal disease and began receiving dialysis. Despite mild dementia, her daughter and physician observed that she had a reasonably good quality of life, enjoyed a variety of activities, and tolerated the dialysis well.

In the last 3 years, however, Mrs. Jones' cognitive ability has declined markedly. Now she only occasionally recognizes her daughter and is entirely dependent for her activities of daily living. She is mostly mute, except when she cries out in pain or fear, and shows signs of pleasure only when being spoon-fed or when listening to an accordion player who visits the home every month. Throughout this time, her daughter has continued to visit frequently and has always appeared to have her mother's best interests in mind.

Recently, each trip to dialysis has become an ordeal for Mrs. Jones. She resists getting on the transport gurney and fights the introduction of the arteriovenous catheters. A medical work-up reveals no new underlying illnesses to account for this change in behavior, and

continued on page 4

Case History *continued from page 3*

her physician ascribes her response to progressive dementia. The nursing home director, Dr. Andrews, begins to believe that dialysis is more of a burden than a benefit for Mrs. Jones. Furthermore, the director feels that dialysis may be a waste of resources for someone with such a poor "quality of life."

Without dialysis, Mrs. Jones would surely die in several weeks. Dr. Andrews discusses the situation with Mrs. Jones' daughter, who requests that her mother continue to receive dialysis. She argues that "mom was always a fighter who loved life" and that she deserves to have "everything" done for her. Besides, she observes, Medicare pays for the treatments, so the nursing home need not worry about reimbursement.

Commentary

Both Mrs. Jones' daughter and Dr. Andrews are concerned about the patient's welfare. Nevertheless, they disagree over what course of action is ethically appropriate. Is Mrs. Jones' dialysis a case of futile care, as the nursing home director believes? Or should she receive "everything," as requested by her daughter? And what about the issue of wasted resources? In today's constrained health care environment, should expenditures such as dialysis for demented patients be limited? Each of these questions deserves further exploration.

While many agree that patients have a clear right to refuse unwanted life-sustaining treatments, there is less consensus about the right to demand those same life-sustaining treatments once a dismal prognosis has been made. Many physicians, conflicted about providing this care, are looking for guidance on the question of "futility." To clarify the discussion, some have defined the word in qualitative, quantitative, and physiological terms (1,2).

Qualitative futility means that applying the treatment will not improve the patient's quality of life, which is already considered unacceptably poor. The obvious problem with a qualitative definition of futility is that patients (or their surrogates) and physicians may disagree on exactly what constitutes a poor quality of life (3).

The concept of *quantitative futility*, on the other hand, does not consider quality-of-life issues. Under this definition, a numeric probability of survival—less than 1 in 1000, for example—is used to decide which treatments can be considered futile and should not be offered because the patient is unlikely to survive, even with the intervention (1). This view accords physicians much discretion, including authority to make unilateral treatment decisions. Some disagree with this definition, however, stating that determining such a cutoff is value laden and can still result in serious disagreement between patients and physicians.

Finally, *physiological futility* has been suggested to define situations in which it is impossible for the intervention to benefit the patient at all (2). Under this type of definition, prolonged artificial hydration and nutrition for a patient confirmed to be in a persistent vegetative state would not be futile because the patient would physically benefit from such treatment, but performing a lung transplant for someone with widely metastic lung cancer would be futile. While nearly everyone agrees that in cases of physiological futility physicians are not obligated to provide treatment, there is less consensus about what to do in cases of qualitative or quantitative futility, when the patient or surrogate chooses continued treatment.

Rather than arguing about futility, perhaps a better way to approach a case like that of Mrs. Jones is to frame the discussion around her goals for care. If her daughter and Dr. Andrews can agree on the overall goals, then treatment decisions, such as dialysis, can be evaluated in light of these goals. For example, is comfort or longevity the primary goal? And how much discomfort does Mrs. Jones' daughter believe her mother would be willing to suffer in order to lengthen her life? Renal dialysis will achieve the goal of keeping the patient alive, but it will not achieve the goal of improving her quality of life or restoring her cognitive function. Furthermore, the price of longevity may be having to fight or sedate a combative patient.

Oftentimes, discussing a dilemma by focusing on goals will help resolve differences. It turns out that the problem is not so much a true disagreement as a misunderstanding over what goals are and are not achievable.

Speaking about goals also helps put requests that "everything" be done into a proper context. In fact, such requests ought never be left unexplored. As with futility, "everything" is only a useful statement in reference to some goal. Would this daughter really want her mother to undergo a screening persantine-thallium test, cardiac catheterization, and bypass surgery for any detected lesions?

The nursing home director raised the question of appropriate resource allocation. Could the money being spent on dialysis of this demented patient be better used to treat more functional patients? This is certainly a valid policy concern; however, the American College of Physicians (ACP) Ethics Manual states that "decisions on resource allocations must not be made in the context of an individual patient-physician encounter but must be part of a broader social process" (4). Making decisions at the community level is thought to help ensure fairness because decisions are less likely to be arbitrary, and there is a greater likelihood that money saved will be channeled into more appropriate needs.

On the other hand, some who have proposed definitions of futility and frameworks for thinking about the issue maintain that cost not be a consideration in medical futility determinations, and that the focus be the likelihood and quality of the expected benefit (5).

Given this background, how ought the physician facilitate decision-making for an incompetent patient? First, Dr. Andrews should determine whether Mrs. Jones has a written advance directive that would direct providers toward her wishes and/or a surrogate decision-maker. In this case there is none. Dr. Andrews should also explore whether Mrs. Jones discussed her wishes with her daughter or someone else. She should then identify an appropriate decision-maker. In this case, although the daughter was not formally appointed as Mrs. Jones' surrogate decision-maker, she has acted in that role without question until now and seems to have her mother's best interest in mind. Physicians should be aware that laws and processes for determining who should be a surrogate decision-maker vary from state to state.

In cases where the patient has not left an advance directive, physicians and surrogates should first try to make a decision based on substituted judgment. By taking into account what is known of the patient's values, goals, and previous choices, physicians can make a decision that best approximates what they believe would have been the patient's decision. In cases where such values and preferences are unknown, surrogate decision-makers must base their decision on what they believe to be in the patient's best interests. This is done by taking into account current and projected quality of life according to the patient's perspective. When using either of these standards, physicians must be aware that local law may be relevant to decision-making regarding treatment (4).

By focusing on the quality of communication between the physician and surrogate, much more can be done to resolve the dispute and achieve an ethically acceptable result (6). Discussion between Dr. Andrews and Mrs. Jones' daughter must be open and frank. The physician should acknowledge that the daughter has suffered because of the loss of her mother as she knew her and give her support. Dr. Andrews should explore the daughter's goals for care for her mother, outline a realistic prognosis (e.g., continued cognitive decline), and present various treatment options. In discussing the option of withdrawing dialysis, the physician should address the daughter's potential fears about pain and discomfort and reassure her that withdrawing dialysis does not mean withdrawing care. Dr. Andrews should outline the specific palliative measures that would be used and explore exactly what Mrs. Jones' daughter means when she says she wants "everything" for her mother, and what limits, if any, the daughter would set. Finally, the physician needs to identify any remaining areas of true disagreement. For example, even after being educated about all the options and thinking about the goals of care, Mrs. Jones' daughter may assert that she is acting on her mother's wishes or place greater value than Dr. Andrews on her mother's present quality of life.

Through such communication, most disagreements can be resolved. In this particular case, the patient's own actions may end dialysis. If she continues to actively refuse the procedure, it would seem untenable to sedate Mrs. Jones and fight her 3 times a week for 4 hours of dialysis. If the patient's daughter witnessed these episodes, she would most likely agree to discontinue the intervention. However, if a true disagreement remained in this case, the medical director should not withdraw dialysis unilaterally.

Perhaps the most important lesson to take home from this case is that better advance planning may have prevented this dispute. These issues could have been addressed when Mrs. Jones was first admitted to the nursing home and was still perhaps competent to make decisions. The federal Patient Self Determination Act requires nursing homes to ask prospective residents or family members if advance planning has been discussed and to inform patients of their right to identify their preferences for care in advance. The law does not, however, require individuals to do advance planning.

While a specific therapy such as dialysis may not have been anticipated, a discussion that focused on the patient's overall goals of care would have provided the physician and family members with a better idea of the patient's wishes. In fact, when dialysis was initiated, it would have been useful to outline the goals of therapy and to agree upon when the burdens of the intervention would no longer be worth the benefits of prolonging Mrs. Jones' life.

A similar version of this case study was originally published in ACP Observer in March 1997.

REFERENCES

1. Schneiderman LJ, Jecker NS, Jonsen AR. Medical futility: its meaning and ethical implications. Ann Intern Med. 1990;112:949-54.
2. Truog RD, Brett AS, Frader J. The problem with futility. N Engl J Med. 1992;326:1560-3.
3. Youngner SJ. Who defines futility? JAMA. 1988;260:2094-5.
4. American College of Physicians Ethics Manual, 3rd ed. Ann Intern Med. 1992; 117:947-60.
5. Jecker NS, Schneiderman LJ. Futility and rationing. Am J Med. 1992;92:189-96.
6. Dunn PM, Levinson W. Discussing futility with patients and families. J Gen Intern Med. 1996;11:689-93.

ANNOTATED BIBLIOGRAPHY

American Medical Association Council on Ethical and Judicial Affairs. Medical futility in end-of-life care. JAMA. 1999;281:937-41.

For futility determinations, the AMA recommends health care institutions adopt a policy on medical futility that incorporates a fair process approach. This process should include steps to facilitate deliberation and resolution, determine alternatives where differences are not resolvable, and reach closure.

Cantor MD, Braddock CH, Derse AR, et al. Veterans Health Administration National Ethics Committee. Do-not-resuscitate orders and medical futility. Arch Intern Med. 2003;163:2689-94.

The focus here is on the patient or surrogate decision-maker who wants cardiopulmonary resuscitation to be attempted when the physician believes that resuscitation efforts would be futile. The authors conclude that conflicts over do-not-resuscitate orders and medical futility should be resolved under a policy that uses a defined and fair process addressing specific cases and includes multiple safeguards, not one that defines futility in the abstract.

Fine RL, Mayo TW. Resolution of futility by due process: early experience with the Texas Advance Directives Act. Ann Intern Med. 2003;138:743-6.

In 1999, Texas became the first state with a law providing a due process mechanism for resolving end-of-life care disputes, including those over medical futility. This article reviews the experience of a large tertiary-care teaching hospital with the law.

Youngner SJ. Who defines futility? JAMA. 1988;260:2094-5.

A discussion about the issue of physician decision-making in circumstances involving the use of futile, life-sustaining interventions.

2

Should Doctors Treat Their Relatives?

Commentary by James A. Tulsky, MD, Miriam Shuchman, MD, and Lois Snyder, JD
Case History by Richard J. Carroll, MD

Case History

A 73-year-old woman with a history of hypertension, deep vein thrombosis, gout, and degenerative arthritis calls her son. He is a physician, and she is seeking medical advice. She tells him, "My physician is on vacation and my gout is acting up. I've used ibuprofen in the past and it isn't helping that much. Dr. Smith [her primary care physician] had prescribed another medicine that worked great. I think it was colchicine."

Her son suggests she call the physician covering for Dr. Smith to discuss her situation and, if appropriate, obtain a prescription to renew her medication. She insists her son call the prescription in because "You went to medical school and know my situation better than some doctor on call."

He reluctantly calls in the renewal prescription. But he insists she follow-up with someone else as soon as possible. Fortunately, she is seeing her orthopedic surgeon in 2 days for her arthritis. "He doesn't know anything about gout," she replies, but she agrees to allow him to look at her foot.

Later that week, she calls her son at home. "Well, you were wrong. It wasn't gout but some sort of cellulitis, and now I'm on two different antibiotics." She also insists her son discuss the sequence of events with Dr. Smith as soon as possible.

Commentary

Most physicians periodically provide medical care to their family members and significant others (1-3). Some provide care to friends, employees, and even themselves. There are often good motivations for these practices, and often no apparent difficulties arise. In some instances, however, there may be significant problems, especially if substandard care is provided. What is the nature of the patient-physician relationship in these instances and how does it affect patient care?

Scenarios range from the doctor who performs an ear exam on her 5-year-old son to determine whether he has otitis, to the doctor who does elective abdominal surgery on his wife. These situations occur for several reasons: Family members commonly request care from doctors who are related to them (3). Physicians want to be available to their families, and they may feel obliged to offer their clinical expertise. Physicians may be embarrassed when their family members bother a colleague for what appears to be a simple problem, or they may intervene in the care of a family member because they disagree with his or her clinician (4). And, finally, it is often more convenient, or less expensive, for the physician family member to provide a service rather than for another doctor to be consulted (1).

Many medical societies have policies on whether doctors should treat their families and significant others. For example, the American College of Physicians (ACP) Ethics Manual strongly discourages, but does not prohibit, physicians from treating family members, limiting such situations to those of necessity and cautioning that the patient be transferred to the care of another physician as soon as practicable (5). The American Medical Association (AMA) has a similar position regarding immediate family members. It adds that there are situations in which family members can provide routine care for short-term, "minor" problems (6). No examples are cited, however, and this exception could swallow the rule. The AMA does specify that doctors should write prescriptions for controlled substances for themselves or immediate family members only in emergencies (6). The Canadian Medical Association says that treatment of family members should be limited to minor or emergency care or instances when another physician is not available (7).

John La Puma and E. Rush Priest have posed a series of questions doctors should ask themselves when they are considering providing care for family members. They believe that individual physicians, arriving at personal answers to these questions, will make appropriate decisions about care (8). While these questions are well directed, caring for family members is not only a personal issue but one the profession should acknowledge and manage.

Several problems can arise when physicians care for their relatives. When the patient is a relative, the informal nature of the situation may result in compromised care at any of the different steps in the clinical encounter, including history-taking, physical examination, diagnosis, treatment, and follow-up.

Medical histories in these circumstances are often incomplete or assumed. Physicians may find it difficult to ask family members sensitive questions about drug use, sexual practices, or other highly personal issues; alternatively, patients may be uncomfortable disclosing this information to a relative.

Physicians may omit or abbreviate physical examinations performed on family members, or they may go beyond their area of expertise. In some cases, the relative lives far away and cannot easily be seen by the physician; in other cases, the physician performs the examination without the proper instruments. Additionally, the unease caused by physical intimacy may distract a doctor who needs to probe a parent's abdomen or axilla. Performing a mental status exam on a close relative may be even more difficult than examining the relative's body.

Some have argued that treating family members and other intimates is unwise because emotional involvement interferes with a physician's ability to be objective (2). Such a loss of objectivity can affect diagnostic work-ups. To exclude all possibility of disease, some physicians obtain more tests on relatives than might be done in similar cases for other patients. Conversely, other doctors are less likely to recommend an invasive procedure that could be painful for a relative.

Diagnostic reasoning may also be faulty. For example, physicians might be unwilling to consider a diagnosis of cancer in their spouses. And physicians may alter treatment plans unwisely when they shorten therapies to spare their relatives a hospital visit.

Confusion about what should constitute a patient-physician relationship may influence the doctor to be particularly informal, and this too can compromise care. Physicians may fail to record their encounters, so there may be no documentation and no chart to consult (1). In sum, in the clinical treatment of a family member, or intimate other, doctors are prone to omissions, abbreviations, and informalities that compromise care and can harm patients.

The physician's professional relationship with his or her patients is based on fiduciary responsibility. Family relationships, by contrast, are based on love. Because a clinical encounter with a family member is not part of a typical patient-doctor relationship, physicians caring for family members may tend to ignore standard guidelines, such as respecting a patient's right to decide about treatment, informing the patient about the risks and benefits of treatment and the alternatives, telling patients the truth, and respecting confidentiality. A doctor might withhold the truth regarding a diagnosis from a parent, whereas she would tell the truth if the patient was not related to her. Another doctor might breach the confidentiality of a patient who is a relative. William Spaulding cites the case of a surgeon who told a newspaper reporter about a patient he had operated on. The patient was a relative who had not given him permission to discuss her case (9)!

The care delivered by a physician family member may be minor: an endometrial biopsy, a prescription for a diuretic, or the confirmation of a presumed diagnosis as illustrated in our Case History. Usually, these acts will not lead to unfortunate outcomes. But even simple cases raise potential problems. In this case, which was not an emergency, the physician/son should have stuck by his initial advice that his mother seek care from the covering physician.

How should the profession determine which type of care is ethically and medically acceptable? The most defensible situations are those in which doctors can quickly act within their area of expertise to solve an immediate problem that does not require new medical evaluation. For example, if someone on a trip loses luggage that contains medications, it would seem acceptable for a physician-family member who is on the trip to refill the medications. Slightly less defensible is the situation in which a family member presents with complaints of a simple problem that is identical to a previously treated problem. This person knows the treatment needed and merely wants to avoid the inconvenience of visiting another doctor. In these two situations the physician-relative is "filling in" until the patient's primary doctor is available. However, as our Case History illustrates, avoiding inconvenience for a family member can result in mismanagement and a potentially serious negative outcome.

Less clear is caring for the family member with a new medical problem. If the problem is relatively simple, the services required might be as minor as performing a limited physical exam or prescribing some drugs. However, if the new medical problem is complex, it is harder to justify delivering the care unless the problem is in one's area of expertise, the care required is restricted to minor services, or, especially, if no one else is available to deliver the care. Finally, there are services that seem unacceptable to offer to any intimate or family member, such as acting as the person's primary medical provider, performing major surgery, or acting as the person's individual family psychotherapist.

If it becomes necessary to treat a family member, physicians should consider the following:

In deciding whether a patient is too much of an intimate to treat, the type of relationship is less important than one's emotional closeness. A close friend may be as much of an intimate as one's sibling, child, parent, or significant other. At issue is whether the physician's closeness to the individual obscures the ability to be objective. If this is unclear, the patient should consult with another physician.

Physicians should remind family members that they can provide access to the system and advocacy without directly treating the patient. Many family members prefer advice and referral to another trusted physician over a relative's hands-on care but may not be willing to say so.

Physicians must consider whether the service required falls within their area of expertise. If a request is significantly outside a physician's professional specialty area, the likelihood of a misdiagnosis or incorrect treatment increases.

Physicians contemplating treating family members should carefully assess the limitations of the medical setting. Whenever possible, care should be delivered in the standard practice environment. If the setting is unusual, physicians must be sure that this alternative environment does not compromise quality.

When care is given to family members, physicians should keep records and communicate with the individual's primary physician. Notes on the care of a family member should be accessible and shared with other caregivers. When there is a bad outcome, cases involving family members are appropriate for discussion at morbidity and mortality rounds and other similar forums.

Physicians will always encounter requests for care from their own family members and significant others. We need to acknowledge that in some cases answering these requests directly can result in strained family relations, as well as compromised medical care and patient-physician relationships. Often, the most caring and professional response one can offer is to help the person negotiate the health care system, leaving direct medical care to others. By refusing to be your brother's doctor, but assuring him that you will advise him, you may most rigorously fulfill the commandment to be your brother's keeper.

A similar version of this case study was originally published in ACP Observer in January 1999.

REFERENCES

1. Dusdieker L, Murph J, Dungy C, Murph W. Who provides health care to the children of physicians? Am J Dis Child. 1991;145:391-2.
2. Gartrell NK, Milliken N, Goodson WH, et al. Physician-patient sexual contact: prevalence and problems. West J Med. 1992;157:139-43.
3. La Puma J, Stocking CB, LaVoie D, Darling CA. When physicians treat members of their own families: practices in a community hospital. N Engl J Med. 1991; 325:1290-4.
4. McSherry J. Long-distance meddling: do MD's really know what's best for their children? CMAJ. 1988;139:420-2.
5. American College of Physicians. Ethics Manual, 4th ed. Ann Intern Med. 1998; 128:576-94.

6. American Medical Association. Code of Medical Ethics: Current Opinions. 1996-97.
7. Code of Ethics of the Canadian Medical Association. CMAJ. 1996;155:1176A-1176D.
8. La Puma J, Priest ER. Is there a doctor in the house? An analysis of the practice of physicians' treating their own families. JAMA. 1992;267:1810-2.
9. Spaulding WB. Should you operate on your own mother? The Pharos. 1992; summer:23-6.

ANNOTATED BIBLIOGRAPHY

American Medical Association Council on Ethical and Judicial Affairs. Opinion 8.19, Self-Treatment or Treatment of Immediate Family Members. Code of Medical Ethics: Current Opinions. Chicago: American Medical Association. 2000; 92.

> *Except in emergency or isolated settings, physicians generally should not treat themselves or members of their families. Professional objectivity and care may be compromised due to the physician's personal feelings. Sensitive areas of medical history or parts of a physical exam may be overlooked to avoid feelings of embarrassment.*

La Puma J, Priest ER. Is there a doctor in the house? An analysis of the practice of physicians' treating their own families. JAMA. 1992;267:1810-2.

> *Assists clinicians who are asked to treat their family members by posing various questions, along with standards and solutions for each.*

La Puma J, Stocking CB, LaVoie D, Darling CA. When physicians treat members of their own families: practices in a community hospital. N Engl J Med. 1991;325:1290-4.

> *Study reveals that many physicians reluctantly treat and diagnose family members when they want to decline to provide care.*

Schneck SA. "Doctoring" doctors and their families. JAMA. 1998;280:2039-42.

> *Several management approaches to treating other physicians and family members are offered. Various factors that may pose problems are discussed, followed by ten suggestions to help physicians handle the role of "doctor's doctor."*

3

When Patients Want Alternative Therapies

Commentary and Case History by Richard J. Carroll, MD

Case History

A 47-year-old man comes to your office with classic angina pectoris. Although you don't have information on his cholesterol levels, you know that he is nondiabetic, normotensive, and a former smoker with a positive family history of coronary disease. The patient eventually undergoes angiography. Coronary artery disease is found with a 90% lesion in the left anterior descending artery and nonobstructive plaque in his remaining coronary arteries. A coronary stent is successfully placed, and the patient sees you in follow-up.

After successfully completing cardiac rehabilitation, his total cholesterol is greater than 300 mg/dL with an LDL cholesterol of 230 mg/dL, well above the 100 mg/dL suggested by guidelines from the National Cholesterol Education Project. Even after appropriate dietary changes and weight loss, the patient's cholesterol remains elevated, so you suggest cholesterol-lowering therapy, specifically an HMG Co-A reductase inhibitor.

"You know, Doctor, I'm not much for medicines," the patient states. "Isn't there another way?" You discuss the sequential steps of diet and weight loss you've already initiated. You also explain the scientific data available for this class of medicine, including improved survival when used for the secondary prevention of coronary disease. "That's fine," the patient replies, "but I've read quite a bit about chelation therapy and would prefer to try that first." Although there are alternative treatments that have value, research confirms your thoughts that chelation therapy can be harmful and that there is no evidence of its effectiveness.

continued on page 16

Case History *continued from page 15*

When the patient returns after 4 months of undergoing chelation therapy 3 times a week, his LDL cholesterol remains elevated at 227. Despite your recommendations against chelation therapy and the patient's own experience with its ineffectiveness, he agrees to take the reductase inhibitor only if he can continue with chelation therapy.

Commentary

Chiropractic, chelation, high-dose vitamins, and herbal therapies such as St. John's wort and *Ginkgo biloba* are among the myriad of "alternative" treatments currently enticing and perplexing patients and physicians alike. With approximately $13 billion a year being spent in the United States on these therapies, there must be reasons why patients seek out and use these remedies in addition to—or instead of—conventional medicines (1).

Dealing with the issue has certainly become a challenge for physicians. What constitutes an alternative therapy, and why are such therapies so popular? From a practical and ethical perspective, how should practitioners advise patients who use these methods or preparations? What are our responsibilities to know and inform patients about these therapies?

Alternative therapies, as they have become known, can range from innocuous family remedies to unproven but potentially promising remedies to harmful and ineffective treatments. Many physicians take issue with the term "alternative," feeling it gives a degree of legitimacy to therapies that may or may not be effective. For example, in conventional medicine, alternative usually refers to options within generally accepted medical practices, such as medical vs. surgical therapy for coronary artery disease. One common definition of alternative medicine refers to therapies not widely taught in medical schools, not generally used in hospitals, and not typically reimbursed by medical insurance companies (1). More than 50 medical schools in the United States now offer courses in alternative medicine.

At its methodology conference in 1995, the recently established National Institutes of Health Office of Alternative Medicine adopted a definition of complementary and alternative medicine (CAM): "A broad domain of healing resources that encompasses all health systems, modalities and practices and their accompanying theories and beliefs, other than those intrinsic to the politically dominant health system of a particular society or culture in a given historical period. CAM includes all such practices and ideas self-defined by their users as preventing or treating illness or promoting health and well-being. Boundaries within CAM and between the CAM domain and the domain of the dominant system are not always sharp or fixed" (2).

Because data suggest that a large number of patients already use these therapies, it is the physician's responsibility to inquire about their use in a neutral, nonthreatening manner and to elicit this information in the context of the patient-physician relationship. We need to know what else our patients are taking or doing in order to prescribe conventional treatments safely and effectively. Just as we ask about nonprescribed medicines, such as over-the-counter medicines, we should ask about other modalities patients may be using in addition to—or instead of—conventional methods. Obtaining this information in a respectful manner recognizes patients' roles as partners in their medical care. The key is asking questions in a nonjudgmental way to obtain information necessary to treatment. How physicians respond to the answers can also determine how honest the patient will be with future inquiries.

Once the discussion has been initiated, the physician should find out why patients may be seeking or using alternative therapies and what benefits they hope to obtain. David Eisenberg has summarized the diverse reasons patients explore alternative therapies (3):

"1. They seek health promotion and disease prevention; 2. Conventional therapies have been exhausted; 3. Conventional therapies are of indeterminate effectiveness or commonly associated with side effects or significant risk; 4. No conventional therapy is known to relieve the patient's condition; and 5. The conventional approach is perceived to be emotionally or spiritually without benefit." Understanding these reasons should help physicians structure discussions regarding alternative therapies in a manner that addresses the patient's specific needs.

Physicians should also ask patients about their understanding of, and experiences with, alternative and conventional therapies. This line of questioning can lead to a discussion about why we base our recommendations on available scientific evidence. We should be able to share with patients the data that exist for the therapies we recommend. In addition, physicians should be willing to help research, within reason, alternative therapies about which patients may have questions.

Helping research such therapies shows patients that we are willing to work with them to achieve their best possible health care. It also shows that we are open-minded and willing to learn, and it demonstrates to patients the systematic approach we use to evaluate both conventional and alternative therapies, which is the foundation of medical treatment and advances. By understanding what data are available, within the limitations of our busy practices, we can act as educated patient advocates by pointing out any shortcomings or misinformation to patients.

However, when discussing alternative medicine with patients, we must be careful not to overstep our level of expertise. If we don't know anything about an area or practice, we shouldn't provide an opinion or misinformation. For example, a patient might interpret a casual remark such as "It probably can't hurt you" as a recommendation to try something.

We should also be careful to structure these discussions in scientific, not emotional, terms. We may emphasize that testimonials are not adequate evidence, but we should also be prepared to defend our own methods of practice when less than ideal data exist. We should be willing to admit that what we offer may not be perfect, and that alternative approaches may have benefits of which we may not be aware. By framing the discussion in an atmosphere of openness, honesty, and intellectual curiosity, we convey to patients that their well-being is truly our primary concern.

In counseling the patient in the above case study, it may be helpful to use a classification system to frame the discussion. This system can be used for any therapeutic modality—alternative or conventional—because it is based upon the level of evidence available regarding its effectiveness and use. John Renner has proposed the following classification scheme (4):

Quackery. These therapies are marketed and claims are usually offered as testimonials that are not documented or based on a reasonable pathophysiological rationale or valid evidence of efficacy. Quackery exploits patient fears or desires, though well-informed patients sometimes desire this course, as in the present case.

Folklore. This refers to a class of preparations based on family tradition that is handed down through generations. These remedies are often used in conjunction with conventional medicine to treat minor illnesses. Although not researched, they are also not marketed, and public claims are not made. Occasionally, folklore begins to be marketed aggressively. At that time, clinical trials should be performed to determine if the remedy has therapeutic value.

Unproven or Untested. These therapies are not based on scientific evidence; therefore, no judgment can be made about their safety or effectiveness. Many accepted therapies could fall into this category as unproven or untested in clinical trials.

Investigational Research. Although scientific evidence does not yet exist for these therapies, they are undergoing investigation that uses documented data, accepted research designs for obtaining valid data, peer review of the results, and eventual scrutiny by the scientific community. Researchers must meet ethics committee requirements, and and informed consent of patients is necessary to participate in these programs.

Proven. These therapies have been proven effective by some reasonable degree of scientific evidence. These therapies are currently considered valuable in our present state of knowledge and should become part of conventional care.

With these thoughts in mind, how best should we approach the cardiac patient in our case study? The first step is to begin with care, compassion, and understanding. Subsequent steps should include a database search on chelation therapy, an extensive discussion regarding coronary artery disease and the data on secondary prevention, a dialogue regarding the patient's understanding of what conventional therapy can and cannot offer, and a discussion about the patient's expectations regarding chelation therapy. This case is easier than some because readily available data show that chelation is, at worst, nephrotoxic and, at best, has no proven efficacy.

The patient's desire to pursue this treatment was based mainly on an aversion to conventional therapy. He feared coronary artery bypass surgery and was only willing to accept a stent once he saw the angiogram and realized the immediacy of his needs. After the interventional procedure was completed, despite the evidence supporting reductase inhibitors in secondary prevention, he opted for chelation therapy because he lacked data on its effectiveness and explanations regarding its potential harm. The chelation practitioner had provided him with testimonials from many patients who said they had benefited from the treatment, but when asked to back up these claims with scientific data, the practitioner gave the patient literature that focused mostly on the negative consequences of conventional therapy. Such information clearly exploited the patient's fear of the risks of such therapy. Interestingly, the patient initially refused reductase inhibitor therapy because he did not want to "take a foreign substance into his body" and believed chelation with EDTA was a more natural approach. The patient also discounted sound scientific data supporting conventional treatment as nothing more than "what the medical and pharmaceutical industries want you to believe."

After several months of chelation therapy that produced no change in his cholesterol, the patient agreed to try reductase therapy as long as he could continue chelation therapy. While trying to respect his autonomy and avoid abandoning him, the physician continued to follow the patient, and a compromise was reached to monitor possible serious side effects of the chelation therapy. Fortunately, the patient developed no obvious problems and once reductase therapy was initiated, he achieved a desirable cholesterol level.

Medicine is a process in evolution. The science of today may be the disaster of tomorrow (remember thalidomide?), and therapies that practitioners are skeptical of may eventually prove to be useful. The medical community must seek to establish outcome-based standards for *all* treatments.

Labeling something as alternative does not mean it does not have to stand up to scientific scrutiny. However, if efficacy is demonstrated, the conventional medical community should be willing to accept such therapies and make them available to their patients.

An attitude that only one or the other approach is correct is destructive. We must remember that the patient's best interest is most important. With that in mind, all approaches must include a willingness to undergo scientific review on the basis of valid outcomes-based data. Alternative therapies may have profound negative long-term consequences or exciting positive results. In both circumstances, only a systematic scientific review will bring those results to light.

A similar version of this case study was originally published in ACP Observer in July/August 1998.

REFERENCES

1. Eisenberg DM, Kessler RC, Foster C, et al. Unconventional medicine in the United States: prevalence, costs, and patterns of use. N Engl J Med. 1993;328:246-52.
2. Defining and describing complementary and alternative medicine. Panel on Definition and Description, CAM Research Methodology Conference, April 1995. Altern Ther Health Med. 1997;3:49-57 .
3. Eisenberg DM. Advising patients who seek alternative medical therapies. Ann Intern Med. 1997;127:61-9.
4. John Renner, National Council Against Health Fraud, personal communication.

ANNOTATED BIBLIOGRAPHY

Adams KE, Cohen MH, Eisenberg D, Jonsen AR. Ethical considerations of complementary and alternative medical therapies in conventional medical settings. Ann Intern Med. 2002;137:660-4.

This article urges physicians to consider their ethical duties when "recommending, tolerating, or proscribing" complementary and alternative medical (CAM) therapies. It offers a risk-benefit framework for determinations about use of CAM in different clinical situations.

Astin JA. Why patients use alternative medicine: results of a national study. JAMA. 1998;279:1548-53.

A study of the demographics and factors behind patient use of alternative medicine in the United States. Findings show that use of alternative medicine is linked to the patient's education, philosophical outlook on health ("importance of mind, body, and spirit"), and cultural beliefs.

Eisenberg DM. Advising patients who seek alternative medical therapies. Ann Intern Med. 1997;127:61-9.

Presents an approach to discussing the use or avoidance of alternative medical therapies, emphasizing patient safety, medical record documentation, and shared decision-making.

Eisenberg DM, Davis RB, Ettner SL, et al. Trends in alternative medicine use in the United States, 1990-1997: results of a follow-up national survey. JAMA. 1998;280: 1569-75.

Results from a 1997 national survey to study U.S. patient utilization of alternative medicine. The findings support the presumption that alternative medicine use has increased substantially from 1990 to 1997. Alternative medicine has been primarily sought for treatment of chronic conditions, with a trend in increased visits to alternative medicine practitioners and increased expenditures for alternative services.

Studdert DM, Eisenberg DM, Miller FH, et al. Medical malpractice implications of alternative medicine. JAMA. 1998;280:1610-5.

Clarifies some misconceptions about the current rates of malpractice claims for alternative medicine, relates the situations where the physician could be exposed to liability for referrals, and discusses the process courts use to determine malpractice involving alternative medicine practitioners.

Sugarman J, Burk L. Physicians' ethical obligations regarding alternative medicine. JAMA. 1998;280:1623-5.

Similarities and differences in the principles and culture of practice between conventional and alternative medicine are discussed. By using a "principle-based" analysis, the authors demonstrate the physician's professional and ethical obligations regarding alternative medicine through a discussion of respect for persons, nonmalefience, beneficence, and justice in health care.

4

The Ethical Dilemma of Genetic Testing

Commentary and Case History by Robert A. Aronowitz, MD

Case History

Ms. Thomson is a 29-year-old healthy woman who is worried about her risk for breast cancer. Her maternal grandmother died in her early 50s of breast cancer. Her 27-year-old sister was diagnosed with breast cancer 2 years ago and has already had a lumpectomy, nodal dissection, and adjuvant chemotherapy. Her mother's sister died of ovarian cancer at age 50, and her mother's brother, age 60, has recently been diagnosed with prostate cancer. Ms. Thomson's mother, age 49, has refused to get a mammogram or even see doctors, saying that she has little faith that early detection of cancer makes much difference. Ms. Thomson's youngest sister, who is 25 years old, is also worried about her breast cancer risk but has not sought medical attention and has never had a mammogram.

Ms. Thomson has read stories about the breast cancer gene in the local newspapers. The immediate stimulus for her visit was a lecture about breast cancer at the local library hosted by a breast cancer advocacy group. She requests that she be tested for the "breast cancer gene." She already does monthly self-breast exams, gets mammograms every 6 months, and tries to follow a vegetarian diet. She is also worried that her 2-year-old daughter might have the gene. She says she is sure that she has the gene and wants the test only to confirm her suspicions. However, she is unsure what she would do differently if she tests positive for the gene.

Ms. Thomson is the first person to request BRCA1/2 testing from Dr. Jackson, a primary care physician whom she recently selected through her managed care plan. He calls an oncologist colleague who makes some inquiries and tells him about various options with

continued on page 23

22

> ## Case History *continued from page 22*
>
> in and outside research protocols. Ms. Thomson chooses off-site testing through a private laboratory that also provides information packets for physicians and patients and promises to return test results within 2 months. The laboratory requires that affected relatives also submit blood samples. After reading through the information packet, Ms. Thomson signs a form that states that she understands the risks of testing. Her affected sister agrees to testing, and after some cajoling so does her younger sister. Both also agree to sign forms that specify that Dr. Jackson will disclose the results only to the person who was tested. Ms. Thomson's mother absolutely refuses to participate in any aspect of the testing.
>
> As promised, the laboratory delivers the results 2 months after having received the blood samples. Both Ms. Thomson and her sister who has breast cancer test positive for the gene, while the youngest sister is negative. Dr. Jackson asks the entire family to come in for a discussion of the results, but only Ms. Thomson arrives at his office.

Commentary

Neither Ms. Thomson nor Dr. Jackson know how to use the information provided by BRCA1/2 tests, although some groups have begun to offer guidelines (1). There are no good data on the efficacy of intensive screening for breast and ovarian cancer, prophylactic surgery, or any other proposed interventions for women who have genetic mutations. We do not even know the meaning, validity, and reliability of these tests. Already, data about genetic risk drawn from less selected populations have led to reducing the positive predictive values of BRCA1/2 testing (2).

Additionally, there are many reasons to worry about the psychological and economic implications of genetic testing, especially regarding access to health insurance, employability, and privacy. Given this ignorance and these concerns, many groups urge that genetic testing only be carried out in a research protocol, if at all, and that vigorous safeguards of patient confidentiality be implemented (3). But for many others, the genie is already out of the bottle. The test is available, and many women want to know if they carry the "gene" for breast cancer. How might we balance a woman's understandable interest in learning whether she carries one of the known mutations in susceptibility genes with our ignorance of the test's significance, costs, and benefits, as well as the lack of iron-clad safeguards against the misuse of test results? And even if one believes that there should be constraints on, or guidelines for, testing, how will such rules be enforced or even encouraged in our decentralized, free-market, consumer-driven, health care system?

There are no easy answers to these questions. For the immediate future at least, clinicians such as Dr. Jackson and patients such as Ms. Thomson will have to make difficult decisions under conditions of great uncertainty. Internists might best begin by viewing the issues raised by genetic testing as a new but not radically different challenge than that posed by many other screening and diagnostic testing problems in primary care. Experienced clinicians are already good at trying to place a request for testing in the context of their patients' underlying goals, motivations and fears, degree of risk-aversion, and the familial and other influences on medical decisions.

Returning to Ms. Thomson's situation, Dr. Jackson might begin by asking her what she really wants to know. Many patients, and their doctors, cannot really anticipate what they will do with information as potentially devastating as "having the gene" for breast cancer. Ms. Thomson's fatalistic statement that she is sure that she has the gene seems a defensive and rather thin strategy, belied by her interest in getting tested. She may be motivated as much by her desire to rid herself of the fear of breast cancer, something even a negative test cannot do, or to confirm her worst suspicions, which even a positive test cannot do (in fact it will lead to many new uncertainties). Because coping with fear and uncertainty will be a persistent issue regardless of specific test results and management choices, drawing these motivations from Ms. Thomson and discussing them are as important as assessing whether she is in the "right" risk category for getting the test as recommended by different groups. While Ms. Thomson's strong family history meets many definitions of high risk, the more important and difficult issue is whether her unique goals, motivations, fears, and risk-taking propensities should lead to testing and, if so, to which type of testing.

Because the results of this test affect all the women in her family, it is not just Ms. Thomson's particular situation but her family's that must be considered. Yet Dr. Jackson only has a relationship with Ms. Thomson, and a new one at that. While the test has been carried out on all three sisters, only Ms. Thomson comes in to hear the news. What are Dr. Jackson's responsibilities to Ms. Thomson's sisters? It is highly probable that her mother, who clearly does not want to know, also has the "breast cancer gene." The test results also have implications for Ms. Thomson's 2-year-old daughter. This case points out the coercive aspects of genetic testing since the mother's desire to remain ignorant will be difficult to respect and Ms. Thomson's daughter's values and interests are unknowable. As a result of Ms. Thomson's choice to get tested, both her mother and daughter may face problems down the road with insurance and employability.

This situation has no neat solution. One clinical and policy implication is that families should be involved as much as possible in the decision to test in the first place, and a good faith effort should be made to work out in advance how the information will be shared. Again, what seems most relevant is not spelling out the need for such familial decision making and full consent, which is as obvious as it is unattainable in many situations, but to advocate for systems of care that not only encourage long-term, trusting relationships between physicians and their patients, but also facilitate effective communication between physicians and patients' families.

In addition to these considerations, some believe that there are moral arguments that point to a duty to warn relatives of their genetic risk. As a practical matter, Dr. Jackson may need to encourage Ms. Thomson to explain the potential risks and availability of testing to her mother and eventually to her daughter (although in all probability, scientific advances will lead to very different tests, treatment options, and risk assessments by the time Ms. Thomson's daughter will be in a position to understand the meaning of the current test results).

The case also raises the question of which model of genetic counseling is feasible in the primary care settings in which many women will seek testing and learn their results. Ms. Thomson elected to get off-site testing, and the explanation of risks and benefits was given to her in written materials supplied by the testing laboratory. Her busy primary care physician, who has limited knowledge of breast cancer tests, risks, and risk management, was left to fill in the gaps in the consent process in a brief primary care encounter. This is far from ideal but it would be naive to think that the many reasoned calls for more complete and comprehensive education and consent can be grafted onto routine primary care practice.

In contrast to primary care physicians, genetic counselors have traditionally provided future parents with multiple levels of counseling and education and have told parents that they must make their own decision. This intensive and non-directed model differs from usual primary care practices. Blood pressure checks and cholesterol determination happen in shopping malls, let alone in doctors' offices, and typically without much explicit discussion of the risks and benefits of screening. Policy guidelines in primary care typically suggest particular courses of action. For most tests and treatments in the primary care setting, patients also expect their doctors to give them advice.

Clearly, when facing such uncertainty as to the nature of a new and complex form of testing, it is not unreasonable for a physician to refer a patient to a specialist. However, the primary care physician's role as counselor should not be undermined. One solution is to train primary care physicians in the complexities of genetic information, exhort them to be less directive, and reimburse them for the greatly increased time commitment required for more complete consent. This does not seem feasible given the needs and expectations of most patients, the economic realities of primary care practice, and the lack of any central authority to promulgate and enforce standards. In this case, Ms. Thomson chose what seemed at the time to be the least burdensome testing option and Dr. Jackson concurred in her autonomous decision. But they both may now regret their lack of preparation to deal with the results.

Given present constraints, Dr. Jackson might have served Ms. Thomson better if he had adopted his usual practice in primary care screening decisions, which is to stress and simplify the most essential risks and benefits of the different options, and to offer, if asked, his best assessment of what he might do if he were in her position. He might then have encouraged her to delay testing until more detailed knowledge of risks and consequences develops in the medical literature or to choose testing in a research protocol, so that Ms. Thomson's struggles would have value to others and so that she would receive much more intensive counseling and education.

One thing is clear about the ethical and clinical problems raised by testing for genetic susceptibility to breast and ovarian cancer: they may have been created by basic scientific research and technological innovation, but they will not be solved by them. At the bedside and at the level of health policy and regulation, we will need to find ways of balancing the many uncertainties, limitations, and negative consequences of genetic testing with the potential, but as yet unproven, clinical benefits and the various social and economic interests and psychological factors that make testing so appealing. The sensitive nature of the information most likely will require legislative intervention to protect patients. But for physicians, given current, and likely, future uncertainty, application of the solid principles and practices of long-term doctor-patient relationships will best serve clinicians and patients alike.

A similar version of this case study was originally published in ACP Observer in March 1998.

REFERENCES

1. Hoskins KF, Stopfer JE, Calzone KA, et al. Assessment and counseling for women with a family history of breast cancer: a guide for clinicians. JAMA. 1995;273:577-85.
2. Struewing JP, Hartge P, Wacholder S, et al. The risk of cancer associated with specific mutations of BRCA1 and BRCA2 among Ashkenazi Jews. N Engl J Med. 1997;336: 1401-8.
3. American Society of Clinical Oncology. Statement on genetic testing for cancer susceptibility. J Clin Oncol. 1996;14:1730-6.

Annotated Bibliography

American Medical Association Council on Ethical and Judicial Affairs. Opinion E2.131, Disclosure of Familial Risk in Genetic Testing. Code of Medical Ethics: Current Opinions. Chicago: American Medical Association. 2003.

States that physicians have a duty to protect patient confidentiality, including of genetic information, but that pre- and post-test counseling must include the implications of genetic information for the patient's biological relatives. Discusses the physician's role in the familial aspects of genetic testing.

Hodge JG. Ethical issues concerning genetic testing and screening in public health. Am J Med Genet. 2004;125C:66-70.

The use of genetic testing and screening can improve public health outcomes but also raises ethical, legal, and social concerns. Privacy and informed consent of the patient must be respected, but individual ethical rights have limits. Public health ethics principles justify voluntary genetic testing and screening, and sharing of data for population-based health purposes.

5

Talking About Organ Procurement When a Patient Dies

Commentary and Case History by Vincent E. Herrin, MD, and Peter Poon, JD

Case History

As a third-year medical student, Jane excelled. She thoughtfully researched each of her patients' conditions and was always prepared for rounds. Jane's resident and attending noticed how well she related to each of her patients, particularly a transplant patient, Sam, who had recently received a new kidney.

When the opportunity arose, Jane eagerly attended a special lecture on the ethics of organ transplantation. She was surprised to learn that federal regulations did not allow doctors who were not specifically trained in requesting organ donations to approach a patient's family about donation. According to the regulations, only an organ procurement representative or a trained, designated requester should talk to patients' families about organ donation. Jane suspected that she was not the only person at her medical center unaware of this rule.

Jane's suspicions were later confirmed when she witnessed her resident notify the family of a 42-year-old patient of his unexpected death by heart attack. During the course of the conversation, the resident mentioned that the family should think about organ donation. Jane remembered the resident's exact words to the patient's wife: "I'm sorry to bother you about this, but I'm supposed to ask you about donating your husband's organs."

Jane sensed that the wife felt offended and perhaps even fright-

continued on page 29

Case History *continued from page 28*

ened that the resident would bring up the topic of organ donation. At the same time, Jane could not help but think about Sam, her kidney-transplant patient, and how grateful he was to have received a donated organ.

Jane now realized that neither her classmates nor most of the residents at her medical center had ever received instruction on how to request organ donations from patients or their families. Her resident had recognized the importance of procuring organs, but he wrongly assumed that it was his responsibility to raise the issue with the patient's family. At the end of her rotation, Jane decided to give an oral presentation on the issue of organ procurement, focusing on the new federal regulations.

Commentary

Federal regulations were introduced in 1998 to increase the overall number of organ donations. A study cited in the FR 1998 preamble found that organ donation consent rates were markedly higher when an organ procurement organization (OPO) approached the family about potential donation (67%) than when hospital staff approached the family (9%) (1).

Because of this "overwhelming" statistical evidence, the federal government now requires that the person who approaches the family about organ donation be an organ procurement representative or a designated requester (2). Designated requesters are individuals who have completed a course approved by an OPO on how to approach potential donor families to request organ or tissue donation (3). Physicians are not excluded from becoming "designated requesters." In fact, the government specifically recognizes that physicians may choose to receive training for this role (4).

Before FR 1998 went into effect, most physicians believed that it was their responsibility to broach the topic of organ donation with the families of recently deceased patients (5). The American College of Physicians (ACP) Ethics Manual, 4th ed., which was written before the federal regulations, reflect the traditional view that the potential organ donor's physician "should inquire whether the patient had expressed preferences about donation" (6). As late as 1998, published articles continued to state that "primary physicians are a vital link to encourage patients and families to discuss organ and tissue donation . . . " (7).

This viewpoint rightly acknowledged the benefits of the long-term relationship established between primary care physicians and their patients and families. Ideally, physicians would discuss organ donation with their established patients in the context of advance directives.

Physicians who lack specific training in organ procurement, however, may be unable to provide patients or their families with enough information for them to give informed consent for an organ donation (5). Some physicians may be uncomfortable acting as organ requesters, even if they have a long-term relationship with the patient and family. In addition, as this Case History illustrates, some physicians may not be naturally attuned to the subtleties of timing and communication needed in making organ donation requests (8).

The ethical problem with physician-initiated requests, even by trained physicians, lies in a real or perceived conflict of allegiances (9). On one hand, the physician acts as the principal advocate for his or her patient, caring for medical needs, maintaining vital functions as much as possible, and providing palliative care as life comes to an end. As a designated organ donation requestor, on the other hand, a physician seemingly acts on behalf of potential organ recipients. This conflict may undermine the physician's ethical obligation of beneficence to his or her patient.

The ACP Ethics Manual gives specific directions in certain aspects of the issue: "The potential donor's physician should not be responsible for the care of the recipient nor be involved in retrieving the organs or tissue" (6). Wearing two hats raises suspicion that a physician's attention to the needs of the organ recipient will compromise the care of the donor. Families might even worry that the patient has been declared brain dead prematurely in order to harvest his organs.

Because of the apparent conflict of roles, some have suggested that formal requests for organ donations be made by personnel not directly responsible for the clinical care of the potential donor (9). Others contend that there is in fact no conflict because the physician is merely offering the option of organ donation rather than making a literal request for donation (7). When a patient is in the final stages of dying or has recently died, however, the situation may be too emotionally charged for the family to register the subtle distinction between suggesting and requesting an organ donation.

While physician-initiated requests for organ donation raise ethical concerns, completely removing physicians from the procurement process may be counterproductive. Organ procurement representatives lack the benefit of a previous relationship with the deceased patient's family. Physicians can thus serve as the bridge between the family and the designated requester, emotionally preparing the family for a discussion about organ donation, while at the same time clearly defining their role as an advocate for both the patient and the family.

Such a delineation of roles also ensures that the notification of death is separated from donation requests. Allowing the family time to accept the news of the patient's death is vital. The patient's family must clearly understand that death has occurred, especially in instances where brain death has been established but the patient's body is being technologically supported. Otherwise, disconnecting life support and harvesting organs may be seen as killing the patient.

In one surveyed population, 21% of respondents believed that a patient could recover after brain death (10). The physician has the lead role in helping families understand and accept either a grave prognosis, imminent brain death, or confirmed brain death. An established protocol for communicating about these issues is necessary (11).

Ultimately, if the physician has prepared the way, the job of the organ procurement officer or designated requester will not only be easier but likely more successful, benefiting one or more of the many people in need of organs.

A similar version of this case study was originally published in ACP Observer in February 2000.

REFERENCES

1. 63 Fed. Reg. 33,856, 33,860 (1998), citing Klieger J, Nelson K, Davis R, et al. Analysis of factors influencing organ donation consent rates. J Transplant Coord. 1994;4:132-4.
2. von Pohle WR. Obtaining organ donation: who should ask? Heart Lung. 1996;25: 304-9.
3. 42 CFR 482.45(1)(3) (1998).
4. HCFA Quality of Care Information. Hospital Conditions of Participation for Organ Donation: Questions and Answers, A26. See www.hcfa.gov/quality/4a1.htm.
5. McGough EA, Chopek MW. The physician's role as asker in obtaining organ donations. Transplant Proc. 1990;22:267-71.
6. American College of Physicians. Ethics Manual, 4th ed. 1998.
7. Coolican MB, Swanson MA. Primary health-care physicians: vital roles in organ and tissue donation. Conn Med. 1998;62:149-53.
8. Riker RR, White BW. The effect of physician education on the rates of donation request and tissue donation. Transplantation. 1995;59:880-4.
9. Tolle SW, Bennett WM, Hickam DH, Benson, JA. Responsibilities of primary physicians in organ donation. Ann Intern Med. 1987;106:740-4.
10. The Gallup Organization. The American Public's Attitudes Toward Organ Donation and Transplantation. Conducted for the Partnership for Organ Donation. Boston; Feb. 1993.
11. DeJong W, Franz HG, Wolfe SM, et al. Requesting organ donation: an interview study of donor and non-donor families. Am J Crit Care. 1998;7:13-23.

ANNOTATED BIBLIOGRAPHY

American Medical Association Council on Ethical and Judicial Affairs. Opinion 8.18. Informing Families of a Patient's Death. Code of Medical Ethics: Current Opinions. Chicago: American Medical Association. 2000; 91.

States that attending physicians should not readily delegate the responsibility of disclosing the death of a patient to the patient's family. While at times it may be appropriate for residents to participate in this communication, it is not appropriate to place this duty on medical students.

United Network for Organ Sharing. Policy 2.0. Minimum Procurement Standards for an Organ Procurement Organization. 17 November 2000.

States the policies that provide the minimum procurement standards for an Organ Procurement Organization. Details responsibilities of the OPO that is responding to an organ donor call from a hospital and provides guidelines for certain procedures.

von Pohle WR. Obtaining organ donation: who should ask? Heart Lung. 1996;25:304-9.

Reports successful donation consent achieved by an OPO in 32 of 36 cases compared with 1 success out of 29 cases achieved by physicians.

6

Physician-Assisted Suicide

Commentary by Lois Snyder, JD
Case History by Janet Weiner, MPH

Case History

Ella Washington, age 60, visits Dr. Jones, her internist for the past 20 years, with complaints of nausea, stomach pain, and weight loss. Her work-up reveals pancreatic cancer, with metastases to the liver.

Dr. Jones and Ms. Washington talk extensively about the diagnosis, her poor prognosis, and the lack of curative therapies. In response to her direct question, Dr. Jones says that Ms. Washington probably has less than 6 months to live. He refers her to an oncologist for further advice and schedules another appointment with her a few weeks later to go over the situation.

When Ms. Washington returns, she is accompanied by her husband and son. She has consulted the oncologist and seems to have a clear understanding of her condition. Her family appears supportive as they talk about palliative therapies and home hospice care.

Before leaving, Ms. Washington tells Dr. Jones that she wants to "die with dignity" and needs to be able to take her own life in the least painful way possible when the time comes. She says that she has spoken to her family at length and that they support her decision. She claims that fear of a painful, lingering death will prevent her from enjoying her remaining time. She tells Dr. Jones that she has obtained information from the Hemlock Society on methods of suicide. She asks Dr. Jones to prescribe barbiturates.

Dr. Jones refuses Ms. Washington's request and asks her to return in a few weeks after she consults a psychiatrist to verify that she is not significantly depressed. She complies and then returns to Dr. Jones with the same prescription request. "This is my decision,"

continued on page 34

Case History *continued from page 33*

she says firmly. "We've known each other a long time. I trust you. But if you don't help me, I'll find someone who will, or do it myself. Please don't make this harder on me and my family."

She explains that the security of having enough barbiturates to commit suicide, when and if the time comes, will allow her to live fully and enjoy the present. Dr. Jones is convinced that Ms. Washington is not despondent and is thinking rationally. They agree to meet regularly, and she promises to consult with him before taking her life. Dr. Jones then writes the prescription for barbiturates.

Over the next several months, Ms. Washington enjoys time spent with her husband and son, and renews and reinforces old friendships. She endures intermittent physical and emotional hardships but seems to bounce back from periods of sadness and anger.

Six months after the diagnosis, Ms. Washington becomes much weaker and her nausea and stomach pain grow more constant and intense. Despite extensive efforts to minimize her discomfort, she feels that the immediate future holds what she fears most: increased pain, dependence, and disability. As agreed, she meets with Dr. Jones to inform him that she will soon commit suicide. Two days later, Ms. Washington's husband calls to say that she died at home, after saying good-bye to her family and closest friends.

Commentary

Background

When Dr. Jack Kevorkian enabled Janet Adkins to end her life last year using the "suicide machine" he had set up in his van, attention centered on the fact that he did not have a long-standing doctor-patient relationship with the Alzheimer's disease victim, was not involved in her current care, and was not specially trained in assessing depression. In addition, Mrs. Adkins was not terminally ill.

These issues, though important, deflected discussion from a question that should have already been asked, the foundational question so sharply brought into focus by the case detailed in this article, but common to both cases: Can a physician ever ethically assist a patient who wishes to commit suicide?

The answer over thousands of years of medical ethics tradition has been No. The Hippocratic Oath says No: "I will give no deadly medicine to anyone if asked, nor suggest any such counsel." More recently, the American College of Physicians (ACP) has said No: "Although a patient may refuse a medical intervention and the physician may comply with this refusal, the physician must never intentionally and directly cause death or assist a patient to commit suicide" (1). The American Medical Association has said No: "In assisted suicide . . . the primary purpose of the treatment is to cause death. And that purpose has no role in the professional responsibilities of the physician" (2).

A distinguished panel of physicians, however, recently concluded that "it is not immoral for a physician to assist in the rational suicide of a terminally ill person" (3). Advances in medical technology and compelling cases such as that of Dr. Jones and Ms. Washington require us to look at these issues anew.

Withholding or withdrawing life-sustaining treatment, physician-assisted suicide, and active euthanasia form a spectrum of issues in end-of-life decision-making. Much has been said about the distinctions between forgoing life-sustaining treatment and euthanasia. This commentary, instead, will focus on assisted suicide.

Conflicting 'Goods'

There have always been people who have wanted medicine, through assisted suicide or euthanasia, to help bring about their deaths. That has not changed. Medicine's ability to prolong the dying process in certain circumstances has increased, as has its ability to relieve pain. Not all patients, however, have access to appropriate pain management and supportive care. This may lead some to see suicide as their only option.

Good hospice-type care should be a high priority for all patients. Even though most patients who receive it find that quality terminal care meets their needs, a few, like Ms. Washington, want more control.

The "No's" listed earlier in this commentary reflect the fundamental tenet of medicine that physicians be and be seen as healers and comforters, not agents of death. When physicians cannot heal, however, is life to be sustained at all costs? For example, many physicians agree that once the diagnosis is confirmed, it is not unethical to withdraw the life support of a patient in a persistent vegetative state, based on patient wishes.

Is there, as has traditionally been thought, a clear distinction between omitting care at a patient's request that may or may not result in death and actively and intentionally causing (or assisting to cause) death? Between giving someone the means to end his or her own life and directly ending a life? The preservation of life, the restoration of health, the relief of suffering, and respect for patient autonomy—these four "goods" sometimes conflict. How should they be balanced?

Here, Dr. Jones wants nothing more than to do what is best for a terminally ill patient for whom he has cared for 20 years. He fears the possibility of a botched suicide attempt. Knowing that she does not have much time, Ms. Washington has a clear conception of how she wants to live the remainder of her life. Ms. Washington and Dr. Jones were ultimately able to discuss her views and wishes openly.

In deciding to comply with his patient's wishes, Dr. Jones is doing what he believes will relieve her current and anticipated suffering. In addition, he might say he looked to the principle of patient autonomy as his guide in determining to honor Ms. Washington's request. Ms. Washington had no interest in testing further modern medicine's ability to relieve pain and understood that her strength could not be restored. She foresaw what she believed would soon be a life of increased pain, dependence, and disability.

Sanctity of Life

Physicians are charged to "do no harm." Is there something objectively harmful, or harmful in the eyes of society, about assisting suicide? Ms. Washington maintains that harm will only come to her if Dr. Jones does not help her to live out her remaining time with the peace of mind that will come if she can choose death. She is appealing to Dr. Jones to relieve suffering as she defines it. Can harm be done when a person does not acknowledge or recognize it?

Under a "sanctity of human life" argument, the answer would be Yes. Whether based in religion or on the belief that this principle provides a foundation for social order, "sanctity of life" dictates that life is sacred and should never be taken. Are there exceptions to this rule? Should physician-assisted suicide ever be one?

"Slippery Slopes" and Other Arguments

Those opposing physician-assisted suicide argue further that the potential consequences of such a practice could have adverse effects on health care: "The dedication of the medical profession to the welfare of patients and to the promotion of their health might be seriously undermined in the eyes of the public and of patients by the complicity of physicians in the death of the very ill" (4). Additionally, providing suicide assistance could compromise patient trust in physicians (2).

However, like "slippery slope" arguments, these positions do not address whether it is ever ethical for physicians to provide suicide assistance; rather, they focus on the need for rigorous procedures to safeguard patient rights if assistance is ever to be sanctioned.

This leads us to "slippery slope" arguments. Even if in an individual case—assisting the suicide of a thoughtful, emotionally prepared terminally ill patient such as Ms. Washington—might seem benevolent, what would be the social consequences of the acceptance of this practice? Would patients come to feel they have a "duty" to die? Would this lead to more active and less voluntary forms of euthanasia? What about the risk of error and opportunities for abuse?

These questions are certainly legitimate, but it is possible that they could be satisfactorily addressed by carefully constructed procedures and some kind of oversight of the assisted-suicide process. The primary question remains: *Are there circumstances under which it would be ethical for a physician to provide assistance?*

More Unanswered Questions

More questions remain unanswered: Are some patients requesting assisted suicide because they fear that they will not be allowed to refuse life support when the time comes? Conversely, would demands for assisted suicide create a backlash that would make it more difficult to withhold or withdraw life-sustaining treatment? If assisted suicide were to become accepted, would physicians have less incentive to optimize supportive care?

Public interest in the issue of physician-assisted suicide is deep and pervasive. Opinion polls suggest that about equal numbers favor and oppose it. Clearly the profession, as well as society, needs to continue to discuss the topic and to try to agree on public and professional policy.

In the meantime, physicians cannot be compelled to assist a suicide. And in considering or acting on these issues, physicians should remember that what they consider ethical may conflict with criminal or civil law, which varies from state to state. Physicians may wish to consult with local counsel before taking actions that may have legal consequences for themselves, their patients, and their patients' families.

The Future

The practice of medicine has implications far beyond the examining room. The Hippocratic precept, "first, do no harm," today involves harm done to the patient's rights, as well as to his or her welfare. Respect for patient autonomy, a hallmark of modern biomedical ethics, dictates that physicians uphold the informed treatment decisions of competent patients. The profession's ethical integrity and medicine's obligations to society are threatened, however, when a patient requests the assistance of medicine in order to commit suicide.

Perhaps what is driving the renewed debate about physician-assisted suicide is the rise of patient autonomy seen in the context of treatment refusal. It is a settled question that adult patients (or their surrogates) retain authority for decision-making about health care. But how to define the range of patient decisions that physicians should comply with, and whether requests for physician-assisted suicide fit into that range, is unresolved.

Should physician-assisted suicide be permissible under certain circumstances, a next step beyond the withdrawal of feeding tubes and respirators? Or should it be forbidden under all circumstances? The profession and society need to decide.

A similar version of this case study was originally published in ACP Observer in November 1991.

Editor's note—Since this case study was written, Oregon has become the first and only state in which physician-assisted suicide is legal in certain circumstances. ACP issued a position paper in 2001 opposing the legalization of physician-assisted suicide (see Annotated Bibliography). Chapter 7 revisits this issue.

References

1. American College of Physicians. Ethics Manual, 2nd ed, Part 2. Ann Intern Med. 1989;111:327-35.
2. Orentlicher, D. Physician participation in assisted suicide. JAMA. 1989;262:1844-5, citing the Report of the Council on Ethical and Judicial Affairs of the American Medical Association: Euthanasia. Chicago: American Medical Association; 1989.
3. Wanzer SH, Federman DD, Adelstein SJ, et al. The physician's responsibility toward hopelessly ill patients: a second look. N Engl J Med. 1989;320:844-9.
4. Jonsen AR, Siegler M, Winslade WJ. Clinical Ethics. New York: Macmillan; 1986.

Annotated Bibliography

American College of Physicians-American Society of Internal Medicine. Snyder L, Sulmasy DP, for the Ethics and Human Rights Committee. Physician-assisted suicide. Ann Intern Med. 2001;135:209-16.

In this position paper, the College opposes legalization of physician-assisted suicide. Its routine practice, it is said, would raise serious ethical and other concerns. Legalization would undermine the patient-physician relationship and the trust necessary to sustain it, alter the medical profession's role in society, and endanger the value our society places on life, especially on the lives of disabled, incompetent, and vulnerable individuals. The College, however, remains thoroughly committed to improving care for patients at the end of life.

American Medical Association Council on Ethical and Judicial Affairs. Decisions near the end of life. JAMA. 1992;267:2229-33.

The AMA defines the withholding and withdrawing of life-sustaining treatment, euthanasia, and physician-assisted suicide, discusses them in ethical context, and concludes that the physician must respect the competent patient's decision to refuse life-sustaining treatment. States that physicians must relieve pain and suffering and promote the dignity of patients, but that they should not perform euthanasia or participate in assisted suicide.

Dying well? A colloquy on euthanasia and assisted suicide. Hastings Center Rep. 1992;22:6-55.

A collection of eight articles including international perspectives and a provocative piece by Daniel Callahan, "When Self-Determination Runs Amok."

Miller FG, Fins JJ, Snyder L. Assisted suicide compared with refusal of treatment: a valid distinction? University of Pennsylvania Center for Bioethics Assisted Suicide Consensus Panel. Ann Intern Med. 2000;132:470-5.

On theoretical and practical grounds, this paper defends the position that there is a valid distinction between assisted suicide and refusal of treatment. One of a series of papers developed by the Assisted Suicide Consensus Panel as part of the Finding Common Ground Project of the University of Pennsylvania Center for Bioethics, which appeared in the March 21, 2000 (volume 132) issue of Annals of Internal Medicine (pp 468-99).

Pellegrino ED. Doctors must not kill. J Clin Ethics. 1992;3:95-102; and Compassion needs reason too. JAMA. 1993;270:874-5.

One of the most eloquent considerations of why physicians should not participate in assisted suicide or euthanasia, by one of the founders of modern bioethics.

Quill TE, Cassel C. Professional organizations' position statements on physician-assisted suicide. Ann Intern Med. 2003;138:208-11.

States that there are physicians of good will, deep religious convictions, and considerable palliative care experience on both sides of the debate about legalization of physician-assisted suicide. To respect this diversity, and to encourage the profession to continue to struggle with the genuine dilemmas faced by some patients toward the end of their lives, the authors argue in favor of medical organizations taking a position of studied neutrality on this contentious issue.

Quill TE, Cassel CK, Meier DE. Care for the hopelessly ill: proposed clinical criteria for physician-assisted suicide. N Engl J Med. 1992;327:1380-4.

Three physicians propose clinical standards for when and how to comply with patient requests for physician-assisted suicide.

Wanzer SH, Adelstein SJ, Cranford RE, et al. The physician's responsibility toward hopelessly ill patients. N Engl J Med. 1984;310:955-9; and Wanzer SH, Federman DD, Adelstein SJ, et al. The physician's responsibility toward hopelessly ill patients: a second look. N Engl J Med. 1989;320:844-9.

> *Physician experts convened by the then Society for the Right to Die (now Partnership for Caring) call for flexible care in the treatment of the dying and assert that "it is not immoral for a physician to assist in the rational suicide of a terminally ill person."*

7

Physician-Assisted Suicide Revisited: Comfort and Care at the End of Life

Commentary and Case History by Susan W. Tolle, MD, and Lois Snyder, JD

Case History

Mel Jensen is a 50-year-old man with colon cancer metastatic to the liver who is under the care of his long-time general internist, Dr. Sally Jones. His cancer was diagnosed in October when work-up of hematochezia showed a mass of 15 cm.

In November, he has a sigmoid colectomy and liver nodules are noted. Liver biopsy is positive for metastatic adenocarcinoma. Following surgery, Mr. Jensen functions relatively well at home for several months. In December, he completes a durable power-of-attorney for health care, appointing his wife as his surrogate decision maker should he become unable to make decisions for himself. He repeatedly expresses to Dr. Jones his strong conviction that he wishes to live and fight the cancer as long as there is hope of vigor. But when hope is gone he wants his life to end. He does not want a drawn-out death as his sister recently experienced from breast cancer. His affect is generally upbeat, and his wife and two grown sons are close and supportive.

At an office visit in late January, it is clear that Mr. Jensen is becoming weaker and that oral morphine is no longer fully controlling his pain. Dr. Jones talks with him, and his wife, about enrolling in home hospice care. He agrees and is soon titrated on a self-administered morphine pump to 5 mg/hr. His appetite is poor, but he is physically comfortable.

Dr. Jones remains in close contact and receives frequent calls from Mr. Jensen's hospice nurse. She knows that decisions will need

continued on page 42

Case History *continued from page 41*

to be made within the next few weeks about the possibility of divert-
ing surgery for Mr. Jenson's partial bowel obstruction and the place-
ment of stents for his progressive renal failure. Treatment options are
discussed with Mr. Jensen. He no longer wants anything done to
extend his life, he does not want CPR, he does not want to go back to
the hospital, and he does not want surgery. His pain is now adequately controlled on 25 mg/hr of morphine, but he hates becoming
weak and dependent and asks Dr. Jones to increase the morphine concentration in his pump so he can take his own life by opening it wide.
(With the current concentration and his poor renal function, fluid over-
load might precede respiratory suppression.) With his partial bowel
obstruction, he often vomits his medications and so does not think
he could kill himself with pills. He begs Dr. Jones to order a stronger
solution of morphine.

The family of Mr. Jensen is aware of his request. His sons support
him, but his exhausted wife is ambivalent. She is torn between not
wanting him to suffer and not wanting to hasten his death. The hospice nurse believes her patient can be kept comfortable and finds
assisted suicide morally objectionable. Mr. Jensen continues to
request assisted suicide. What should Dr. Jones do?

Commentary

The Patient and His Request

In the second edition of its Ethics Manual, the American College of Physicians
(ACP) responded with an unconditional No to assisted suicide, stating that,
"although a patient may refuse a medical intervention and the physician may
comply with this refusal, the physician must never intentionally and directly
cause death or assist a patient to commit suicide" (1). An earlier case study in
this series examined the arguments for and against physician-assisted suicide
(see Chapter 6). This chapter revisits the controversy.

In the third edition of its Ethics Manual, the College acknowledged that
there are difficult cases, stating that "open conversations between terminally ill
patients and their physicians about patient needs and values are essential, even
when those conversations include a patient's request for assisted suicide. In most

cases, the patient will withdraw the request when pain management, depression, and other concerns have been addressed. But occasionally the issue of physician-assisted suicide needs to be explored in depth" (2). Is Mr. Jensen's case presented here one of those difficult cases? Dissatisfaction with certain aspects of end-of-life care has been evident in public opinion polls and might also have contributed to the approval of, for example, the physician-assisted suicide referendum in Oregon in 1994. Are patient concerns and the important issues getting addressed? Are they getting addressed here?

The Physician and the Patient: Open Communication

What should Dr. Jones do? Are her initial responses contingent upon her personal values, professional code, and/or state laws regarding assisted suicide? Are there initial steps all health care providers should take regardless of their views on the issue of assisted suicide?

The American Medical Association suggests that "requests for physician-assisted suicide should be a signal to physicians that the patient's needs are unmet and further evaluation to identify the elements contributing to the patient's suffering is necessary" (3). There is general agreement that the initial response to a request for assisted suicide should be further conversation. This begins with a determination in greater depth of the patient's unmet needs, fears, suffering, social circumstances, and pain.

Open dialogue will frequently yield information about unmet needs. Mr. Jensen may fear a time when his pain will not be controlled. He may fear abandonment. He may be depressed. He may be worried about his fatigued wife and the burden he perceives he is placing on her. He may feel alone and scared having not yet thoroughly discussed his wishes and needs. Often through discussions and interventions of a multidisciplinary team the patient's concerns will be satisfactorily ameliorated.

The Physician's Obligation: Pain Relief and Symptom Control

Pain relief must be a high priority of physicians, as long as this is in accord with the patient's wishes (2,4,5). Likewise, the diagnosis and treatment of depression must be given more, and more effective, emphasis in the care of the dying.

Palliative care, the management of pain and symptoms caused by severe illness, includes pain medications and other measures to relieve suffering, as well as counseling and support. However, there have been barriers to effective palliative care. The gradual increase of pain medication in terminal illness to levels that relieve pain is ethically sound, even if a side effect is to shorten life (2).

Some physicians may inappropriately withhold or delay narcotics, fearing that patients will become tolerant to the narcotics or become addicted to them, or because of concern that these drugs will hasten death through respiratory suppression (2). Many hospice proponents maintain, and are making efforts to persuade the public and physicians, that few patients require high doses of pain medication and even they do not become addicted (6). Medicine can benefit from hospice expertise.

Some physicians may not be experienced in methods of pain assessment and control or with interdisciplinary approaches to palliative care. Some pharmacy practices and procedures may also be obstacles (7). Palliative care experts maintain that pain can be alleviated in all but the rarest of cases (7). Better training and continuing education for health professionals, practice guidelines, patient and public education materials, and changes in pharmacy practices can help make that belief a reality.

Health Professionals, Professional Societies, and Diverging Views

In May 1995, the Northern Territory of Australia became the first place in the world to legalize euthanasia. Euthanasia is not legal in the Netherlands, although if established protocols are followed there is agreement not to prosecute. In the United States, no state specifically allowed assisted suicide until Oregon, by popular vote, endorsed physician-assisted suicide in a November 1994 voter referendum, although court challenges barred the implementation of that measure until October 1997.

Even if legal prohibitions are lifted, many health professionals and professional societies oppose assisted suicide. Some health care providers find assisting a patient with suicide morally acceptable when all other modalities have been explored and failed. In Washington, a survey suggested that health care professionals, like the Oregon referendum voters, are nearly evenly split on this issue (8). Thus it is likely that members of any particular health care team will have differences of opinion.

The hospice nurse in the above case believes Mr. Jensen can and should be kept comfortable and finds assisted suicide objectionable. Even if legal and professional prohibitions are lifted, the expression of moral conscience of each individual health care provider should be respected. Dr. Jones has an obligation to ensure that she does not coerce or involve the participation of others in an act they find morally reprehensible. Likewise, consideration should be given to the potential burden placed on family members. Mr. Jensen's wife is not decided, and her current and long-term emotional needs regarding her husband's decision must be considered.

ACP issued a position paper in 2001 opposing the legalization of physician-assisted suicide but continues to probe this issue. The decision to legalize this practice rests with society, not simply the medical profession. Each individual case, however, deserves a respectful hearing and an active effort by the physician to elicit the concerns that led to the patient's request for suicide assistance and to alleviate the patient's distress.

A blanket condemnation of physician-assisted suicide with no consideration of the surrounding issues misses an opportunity to improve the care of a dying patient. Physicians have an obligation to understand the stimulus behind the patient's request and the explore with the patient his or her fear, isolation, suffering, depression, pain, and familial and economic concerns. Society has an unfulfilled obligation to ensure access to hospice-type resources for all dying persons. ACP continues to encourage open conversation, the enhancement of pain relief and symptom control for the dying, and respect for the consciences of all health care providers as we continue to examine the issue of physician-assisted suicide and affirms a professional ethic to improve the care of patients and families facing these issues.

A similar version of this case study was originally published in ACP Observer in September 1995.

REFERENCES

1. American College of Physicians. Ethics Manual, 2nd ed. Ann Intern Med. 1989; 111:254-52, 327-35.
2. American College of Physicians. Ethics Manual, 3rd ed. Ann Intern Med. 1992;117: 947-60.
3. American Medical Association. Council on Ethical and Judicial Affairs. Code of Medical Ethics: Reports, Vol. 5, No. 2. Chicago; 1994.
4. Agency for Health Care Policy and Research. Management of Cancer Pain. AHCPR Pub. No. 94-0592 (Rockville, MD; Department of Health and Human Services, Public Health Service, AHCPR, March 1994).
5. Buchan ML, Tolle SW. Pain relief for dying persons: dealing with physicians' fears and concerns. J Clin Ethics. 1995;6:53-61.
6. Stoddard S. Terminal, but not hopeless. New York Times. 21 August 1991.
7. New York State Task Force on Life and the Law. When death is sought: assisted suicide and euthanasia in the medical context. New York; 1994.
8. Cohen JS, Fihn SD, Boyko EJ, et al. Attitudes toward assisted suicide and euthanasia among physicians in Washington State. N Engl J Med. 1994;331:89-94.

ANNOTATED BIBLIOGRAPHY

American College of Physicians-American Society of Internal Medicine. Snyder L, Sulmasy DP for the Ethics and Human Rights Committee. Physician-assisted suicide. Ann Intern Med. 2001;135:209-16.

In this position paper, the College opposes legalization of physician-assisted suicide. Its routine practice, it is said, would raise serious ethical and other concerns. Legalization would undermine the patient-physician relationship and the trust necessary to sustain it, alter the medical profession's role in society, and endanger the value our society places on life, especially on the lives of disabled, incompetent, and vulnerable individuals. The College, however, remains thoroughly committed to improving care for patients at the end of life.

Buchan ML, Tolle SW. Pain relief for dying persons: dealing with physicians' fears and concerns. J Clin Ethics. 1995;6:53-61.

Finds that pain management for the terminally ill is inadequate. Reviews physician causes of the insufficient use of pain medication and the ethical concepts underlying adequate pain relief.

Conwell Y, Caine ED. Rational suicide and the right to die: reality and myth. N Engl J Med. 1991;325:1100-2.

Two psychiatrists shed some light on the lack of attention given to psychiatric illness in decision-making about so-called "rational suicide."

Foley KM. The relationship of pain and symptom management to patient requests for physician-assisted suicide. J Pain Symptom Manage. 1991;6:289-97.

Maintains that access to expertise in the control of pain, psychological distress, and quality of life must be addressed for the cancer patient.

Miller RJ. Hospice care as an alternative to euthanasia. Law Med Health Care. 1992; 20:127-32.

Reviews the ethical basis for hospice and considers the question, Does hospice care make considerations of euthanasia unnecessary? The author answers Yes.

Miller FG, Fins JJ, Snyder L. Assisted suicide compared with refusal of treatment: a valid distinction? University of Pennsylvania Center for Bioethics Assisted Suicide Consensus Panel. Ann Intern Med. 2000;132:470-5.

On theoretical and practical grounds, this paper defends the position that there is a valid distinction between assisted suicide and refusal of treatment. One of a series of papers developed by the Assisted Suicide Consensus Panel as part of the Finding Common Ground Project of the University of Pennsylvania Center for Bioethics, which appeared in the March 21, 2000 (volume 132) issue of Annals of Internal Medicine (pp 468-99).

New York State Task Force on Life and the Law. When death is sought: assisted suicide and euthanasia in the medical context. New York; 1994.

> *This report reaffirms prohibitions against physician-assisted suicide and euthanasia and calls for better diagnosis and treatment of depression along with better palliative care.*

Quill TE, Byock IR for the American College of Physicians-American Society of Internal Medicine End-of-Life Care Consensus Panel. Responding to intractable terminal suffering: the role of terminal sedation and voluntary refusal of food and fluids. Ann Intern Med. 2000;132:408-14.

> *A small percentage of terminally ill patients receiving comprehensive care reach a point at which their suffering becomes severe and unacceptable despite intense palliative efforts. Some of these patients request that death be hastened. This paper presents terminal sedation and voluntary refusal of hydration and nutrition as potential last resorts in addressing the needs of such patients.*

8

Ethics and Elder Neglect
Commentary and Case History by Janet Weiner, MPH

Case History

Cecilia Griffith, age 80, sustained a right hip fracture that was pinned 6 months ago. Since that time, she has been using a wheelchair. Despite physical therapy, she remains unable to walk, even with the aid of a walker.

Arnold Silver has been the Griffith family's primary care physician for many years. Mr. Griffith died of congestive heart failure about 5 years ago; subsequently, Ms. Griffith moved in with her son Michael, his wife, and their teenage daughter.

Since her hip fracture, Ms. Griffith has seen Dr. Silver monthly. At this month's visit, he is surprised by her generally disheveled appearance and subdued demeanor. He is also surprised to see Michael, because Michael's wife usually brings Ms. Griffith to her appointments. Michael explains that he recently lost his job, and that his wife has taken a temporary job to keep the family afloat.

Upon physical examination, Dr. Silver becomes concerned with a few new findings. Ms. Griffith has a decubitus ulcer on her right hip and smells of urine. She denies being incontinent and says she has been feeling the same as usual. She states that she hasn't been getting out of bed much because she doesn't want to go anywhere.

Dr. Silver, having known Ms. Griffith a long time, senses that something has changed in her living situation. He questions her, without Michael in the room, about the family circumstances. She tells him that Michael is very upset about losing his job and furious that his wife has to go to work. The couple is fighting more than they ever have.

"It sounds like a stressful situation," Dr. Silver remarks. "How does it affect you?"

continued on page 49

Case History *continued from page 48*

"Oh, I try to stay out of everyone's way and not be a burden," Ms. Griffith answers. Upon close questioning, Dr. Silver finds out that Ms. Griffith has not been to physical therapy in about a month. Michael's wife had been Ms. Griffith's primary caregiver, a role that is now being filled by Michael. Given the physical findings, Dr. Silver suspects that Ms. Griffith is not receiving enough assistance with getting out of bed, reaching the bathroom, and personal hygiene. He worries that continued neglect will have irreparable consequences for Ms. Griffith's health and functional status.

"Is Michael able to give you all the help you need throughout the day?" Dr. Silver asks. "Perhaps you need someone else to help you. Would you like me to talk to Michael about it?"

Ms. Griffith becomes agitated and insists that Dr. Silver not bring up the subject with Michael. "He's under so much pressure . . . Don't make it worse. I'm fine and I don't need any help."

What should Dr. Silver do?

Commentary

The issue of mistreatment of elderly people was brought into public view more than a decade ago in a congressional report, "Elder Abuse: An Examination of a Hidden Problem" (1). Since that time, a variety of state laws, health professionals, and social service agencies have tried to address the problem, with varying degrees of effectiveness. For physicians treating elderly patients, the possibility of abuse or neglect poses both ethical and practical dilemmas. This Case History illustrates some of these dilemmas.

Elder mistreatment covers a spectrum of behaviors, from intentional physical abuse to financial abuse to unintentional neglect. Although the incidence and prevalence of elder mistreatment is difficult to measure, a Congressional subcommittee in 1990 estimated that about 1.5 million people (5% of the nation's elderly population) may be victims each year (2).

All physicians with elderly patients should be aware of the signs of elder mistreatment and be able to intervene appropriately. The American Medical Association recently issued guidelines on the diagnosis and treatment of elder abuse that offer physicians guidance on how to recognize and assess mistreatment (3). However, the appropriate course of action for physicians may be clearer in cases of intentional physical violence than in this case, which involves unintentional neglect. Dr. Silver, having known the Griffith family for many years, is convinced that Michael does not mean to harm his mother but is probably overwhelmed by his own difficult circumstances and the extent of his mother's care needs. However, the neglect is not benign; it is already having detrimental effects on Ms. Griffith's health and Dr. Silver must intervene in some way.

This case presents the physician with two fundamental ethical dilemmas: how to balance acting in the patient's best interests with respect for a competent patient's wishes and how to resolve the conflict between the patient's right to confidentiality and the requirements of mandatory reporting laws.

Elderly people have the right to make decisions about their care and about their lives. Age alone, in the absence of other factors causing incompetence, should not be a reason to ignore or supersede a patient's wishes. But in this case, Dr. Silver believes that Ms. Griffith's wishes may not be in her best interests. As such, he should handle this situation as he would other types of disagreements between patients and physicians—with extensive and open discussions. He should ensure that Ms. Griffith understands all her options, and that her decision is not based on fear or coercion. A dependent elderly person, though competent, may feel intimidated by or fear reprisal from her caretaker. Dr. Silver should be sensitive to his patient's perceptions and how they might affect her decision-making. At the same time, Dr. Silver should consider the potential for making the situation worse by possibly leaving his patient open to reprisal or escalation of the mistreatment.

Dr. Silver should determine his next steps using the benchmark of what would be most helpful to Ms. Griffith. His goals should be:

- to help her get the care she needs. Given the complexity of the medical and psycho-social problems facing the family, referrals should be offered to a comprehensive geriatric center, if available, or to social service agencies that may be able to arrange a visiting nurse or home health or respite services. A home health assessment, either by Dr. Silver or a visiting nurse, may clarify the family situation and point out the specific services that would be most useful.

- to preserve their long-standing physician-patient relationship. Dr. Silver should find a way to respect his patient's wishes and keep her trust, while still intervening in some fashion. Perhaps Dr. Silver can ask Michael if he knows how to take care of his mother and if he thinks he needs any help or advice. Dr. Silver should avoid blaming the family or the patient. It may be best to broach the subject with Michael in terms of his mother's new clinical problem rather than in terms of deficiencies in her care. Dr. Silver could say, "Your mother has developed a new medical problem that needs more care than you can give her yourself . . . Let's talk about the options."

- to provide close follow-up and continuing care. Whether or not additional help is accepted, Dr. Silver should maintain close contact with Ms. Griffith and monitor her condition. He should schedule another appointment soon. As Ms. Griffith's primary care physician, he should be her principal point of contact with the medical system and should facilitate a multidisciplinary approach to her health care.

What should Dr. Silver do if the mistreatment continues (or escalates) and Ms. Griffith's condition worsens? To take the scenario a step further: In subsequent office visits, Dr. Silver finds that Ms. Griffith may have developed osteo-myelitis at the site of her ulcer, and the family remains unwilling to accept any help. At this point, Dr. Silver believes that he needs to take further steps to protect his patient's health and considers whether these circumstances fall into the category of reportable abuse and neglect. Is reporting in his patient's best interests? And if he reports the Griffiths to the state, has he violated his patient's right to confidentiality?

Nearly all states have laws that require a variety of health professionals to report suspected elder abuse and neglect to a state agency (usually Adult Protective Services). Considerable debate exists on the effectiveness of mandatory reporting laws for elder abuse. Conceptually, these laws are similar to child abuse statutes in that they are based on the state's power to protect people who cannot protect themselves. But no such reporting requirement exists in the case of non-elderly, competent adults, who have the right to refuse referrals to a state agency. And a recent General Accounting Office study concluded that raising public and professional awareness is a more effective strategy in the identification of cases than are mandatory reporting statutes for elder abuse (4).

Legally, it is likely that a physician is protected from liability if the report is made in good faith. While little case law exists on the subject, it is also likely that a physician's legal duty to report cases of suspected abuse would supersede physician-patient confidentiality requirements (3). However, ethically, the physician must be concerned about how reporting suspected abuse would affect trust and the physician-patient relationship. Practically, the physician must also be concerned about the protective agency's ability to follow up appropriately and the potential for making the situation worse.

Physicians report elder abuse infrequently. One study of physicians in North Carolina documented the perceived barriers to reporting, including confusion about reporting requirements, ignorance of reporting procedures, uncertainty about guarantees of confidentiality, fear of protracted litigation, and cynicism about the state's ability to handle reports (5). Significantly, the study found that physicians who had actually encountered elder abuse had the least confidence in the reporting system.

There is some cause for physician skepticism about the effectiveness of mandatory reporting. State agencies that are charged with investigating elder abuse and providing services to its victims are often chronically underfunded. According to a 1990 Congressional report, states spent just $3.80 per elderly resident annually on protective services, compared with $45 per child annually on protective services (2). Within admittedly limited state budgets for protective services in general, less than 4% on average was devoted to services for the elderly.

Dr. Silver must decide whether to report the situation to a state agency. At what point is he legally required to report? If it is clear that the situation falls under mandatory reporting requirements, Dr. Silver should report it immediately. If it is not clear, Dr. Silver should use his patient's best interests as a standard. Will Ms. Griffith be better off if he reports? Can a state agency offer services that will improve the situation for both the patient and family? Dr. Silver's decision should be informed by an accurate understanding of state law and a knowledge of the process that begins with a report of suspected elder mistreatment. Apart from reporting issues, Dr. Silver should maintain a close connection with the family and continue to provide ongoing medical care. He should creatively use resources such as visiting nurses and respite care, and, if unsuccessful, he should help the patient explore alternative living situations to improve her condition.

A similar version of this case study was originally published in ACP Observer in May 1994.

REFERENCES

1. Select Committee on Aging, U.S. House of Representatives. Elder Abuse: An Examination of a Hidden Problem. Comm. Pub. No. 97-277, April 1981.
2. Select Committee on Aging, U.S. House of Representatives. Elder Abuse: A Decade of Shame and Inaction. Comm. Pub. No. 101-752, April 1990.
3. American Medical Association. Diagnostic and Treatment Guidelines on Elder Abuse and Neglect. Chicago: American Medical Association; 1993.
4. U.S. General Accounting Office. Elder Abuse: Effectiveness of Reporting Laws and Other Factors. Washington, DC: GAO, 1991.
5. Daniels RS, Baumhover LA, Clark-Daniels CL. Physicians' mandatory reporting of elder abuse. Gerontologist. 1989;29:321-7.

ANNOTATED BIBLIOGRAPHY

American Medical Association Council on Ethical and Judicial Affairs. Physicians and family violence: ethical considerations. JAMA. 1992;267:3190-3.

Reviews an ethical duty to diagnose and treat family violence based on the principles of beneficence and non-maleficence. Discusses barriers to intervention, confidentiality, and informed consent. Concludes with recommendations for intervention.

Cammer Paris BE, Meier DE, Goldstein T, et al. Elder abuse and neglect: how to recognize warning signs and intervene. Geriatrics. 1995;50:47-53.

Discusses risk factors and the signs of elder abuse and neglect.

Daniels RS, Baumhover LA, Clark-Daniels CL. Physicians' mandatory reporting of elder abuse. Gerontologist. 1989;29:321-7.

Physicians who were surveyed were concerned about their competence to diagnose abuse, uncertain about reporting laws, and reluctant to report abuse.

Jecker NS. Privacy beliefs and the violent family: extending the ethical argument for physician intervention. JAMA. 1993;269:776-80.

Asserts that family privacy concerns make physicians reluctant to respond to domestic violence. Calls for an analysis of the physician's ethical duties that includes the principle of justice in order to encourage intervention.

Jogerst GJ, Daly JM, Brinig MF, et al. Domestic elder abuse and the law. Am J Public Health. 2003;93:2131-6.

Data were collected on domestic elder abuse reports, investigations, and substantiations in all states and the District of Columbia for 1999. State statutes and regulations pertaining to adult protective services were reviewed. Found 190,005 domestic elder abuse reports from 17 states, 242,430 domestic elder abuse investigations from 47 states, and 102,879 substantiations from 35 states. Significantly higher investigation rates were found for states requiring mandatory reporting and tracking of numbers of reports.

Lachs MS, Pillemer K. Abuse and neglect of elderly persons. N Engl J Med. 1995; 332:437-43.

Defines abuse and discusses prevalence and risk factors for the elderly, clinical evaluation, and management and reporting requirements.

Levine JM. Elder neglect and abuse: a primer for primary care physicians. Geriatrics. 2003; 58:37-40, 42-4.

Finds that factors contributing to misdiagnosis and underreporting include denial by both the victim and the perpetrator, clinician reluctance to report victims and clinician lack of awareness of warning signs. Dependency, on the part of the victim or perpetrator, and caregiver stress are frequent in abusive situations. Concludes that awareness of the risk factors and clinical clues will allow primary care physicians to provide early detection and intervention for elder neglect and abuse.

National Center on Elder Abuse. The National Elder Abuse Incidence Study. Washington, DC: American Public Human Services Association; 1998.

Estimates that approximately 550,000 persons aged 60 years or older experienced abuse or neglect, or both, in domestic settings in 1996.

Part II

THE PATIENT AND THE PHYSICIAN: NON-CLINICAL DIMENSIONS OF THE RELATIONSHIP

Poking and prodding, tests and prescriptions, and other clinical aspects of the direct provision of care are not the only aspects of the patient-physician relationship. The physician's duties and the patient's appropriate expectations extend beyond the laying on of hands, which is itself a problem if not done for clinical reasons.

Part II comprises a diverse sampling of important non-clinical issues that affect the patient-physician relationship: patient requests for particular care, patient refusal to see a recommended specialist, confidentiality and medical record documentation, counseling the impaired driver, what to do and how to discuss the discovery of a physician's mistake made in the course of care, and sexual contact between physician and patient.

9

Direct-to-Consumer Advertisements: How Should You Handle the Pressure?

Commentary by Peter Poon, JD, and Lois Snyder, JD
Case History by Richard J. Carroll, MD, and Lois Snyder, JD

Case History

Thomas Suit, a 38-year-old attorney with a family history of premature coronary artery disease, is talking with his wife at the dinner table. "You know, honey," she says, "with your dad recently dying of a heart attack and all the stress you're under at work, you really should have a checkup. I heard a radio ad about a new painless heart scan where they can tell you whether or not you have heart disease with one quick test."

That week, when Tom sees an ad for a cholesterol medicine, he remembers his wife talking about the radio commercial for the heart scan. The examination is offered at a hospital a few blocks from his office. He decides to have the examination done, if only to make his wife happy. When Tom finds out his insurance won't cover the test, he is aggravated, but he pays for the procedure out of pocket. A few days later, he is confused and frightened when he finds out his test results are "abnormal." He is told to follow up with his private physician.

Tom calls a local internist he has never seen and asks for an immediate appointment to discuss medicines and heart surgery. He is desperate to avoid the fate that befell his father. The physician, however, has no new patient office visits available for 2 weeks.

"If the doctor can't see me today, can I at least get started on that heart medicine that I read about that prevents heart attacks?" Tom asks the receptionist. "My law partner takes it."

When the receptionist tells Tom that he needs to see the doctor first, he insists that he needs the medicine right away. "Can the doctor at least call it into my pharmacy since I have to wait so long to have an appointment with him?" he asks. Finally, the receptionist agrees to squeeze Tom in for an appointment.

Commentary

This Case History illustrates an increasingly common scenario in today's medical practice: patients who suggest their own diagnosis or therapeutic course based on information they cull from print and Internet advertisements and television and radio commercials.

Advertisements for pharmaceutical products and medical technologies such as ultra-fast CT heart scans and new forms of eye surgery are plentiful. The United States is the only industrialized nation that allows prescription drugs to be advertised to consumers through the aforementioned media (1). In 1999, the pharmaceutical industry was expected to spend $1.8 billion on consumer-focused advertising in the United States.

Although direct-to-consumer advertising has become commonplace, the practice still raises many questions (2). Can all consumers understand advertised medical information and apply it to their own conditions? Can advertising be considered a form of education? Does the "information" presented in advertisements change patient expectations of the medical encounter and treatment for the better or for the worse? Does it appropriately influence the prescribing habits of physicians?

Supporters have suggested that consumer advertising offers a number of advantages. They say that it can help educate patients about diseases and identify or treat conditions that might otherwise go undetected. They also point out that because consumer advertising delivers information directly to consumers, it gives them greater autonomy in weighing treatment options. With the information gained from consumer advertising, supporters say, individuals can initiate discussions with their doctors, potentially enhancing the patient-physician relationship. (Approximately 55 million people are said to have talked with physicians in 1998 about prescription drugs they saw advertised [1].) Finally, some supporters argue that consumer advertising can increase competition among pharmaceutical companies, lowering drug costs and increasing access to consumers.

Opponents of consumer advertising, however, point to numerous disadvantages. Because advertisements and commercials are promotional, critics charge, they may encourage increased consumption beyond actual need. In addition, advertisements and commercials are typically so brief that many critics worry that they may not give enough information about risks and benefits, comparable options, and drug interactions.

Consumer advertising can also place undue pressure on physicians to compromise their medical judgment in providing advertised drugs to patients who demand them. One study found that "doctors wrote prescriptions 84% of the time they were asked" (1). If physicians choose to deny a patient's request, they must spend valuable visit time correcting patient misconceptions and misinformation. A final disadvantage of direct-to-consumer advertising, opponents say, is that drug-makers may ultimately increase drug prices to cover advertising costs.

When faced with issues raised by consumer advertising, physicians need to balance two principles of bioethics, namely, beneficence (the duty to promote and act in the best interests of patients and the public health) and respect for autonomy (the duty to protect and foster the patient's free, uncoerced choices) (3). In addition, the autonomy principle requires physicians to adhere to the rules of truth-telling and disclosure (4).

Although these principles are generally accepted as standard for physicians, they could be equally applied to pharmaceutical and other health-related enterprises whose consumer advertisements directly affect potential patients. Thus one could argue that only those advertisements that can be considered in the best interest of the potential patient (those that fully disclose the potential benefits and harms of the advertised product or service and those that ensure informed choice of all available options) should be published or broadcast. The information provided in these advertisements should be data-based, unbiased, and specific to patients' needs. Educating those in need, rather than creating a need, should be the primary purpose and outcome of consumer advertising.

Federal Regulations and the Policy of the American College of Physicians

In response to the growth of direct-to-consumer advertising, the Federal Drug Administration (FDA) has created guidelines for direct marketing of prescription drugs to consumers. The guidelines specify the type of information consumer advertising should include and how the information should be presented.

The federal regulations do not, however, authorize the FDA to pre-screen advertising messages. While pharmaceutical companies may voluntarily submit advertising for pre-clearance, the FDA is authorized to regulate advertising only after it is published.

The Ethics Manual of the American College of Physicians (ACP) states that advertising by physicians and health care institutions is unethical "when it contains statements that are unsubstantiated, false, deceptive, or misleading, including statements that mislead by omitting necessary information" (4). This principle can be applied to health care advertising more broadly.

ACP does not favor promotional messages such as advertising as a way to educate patients (5). Some critics question whether consumer advertising by for-profit drug companies is ever in the best interest of patients or the public. Because consumer advertising is currently allowed in the consumer market, ACP "supports strong regulations and strict guidelines to make such advertising as honest and useful as possible (5)."

Specifically, ACP supports mandatory pre-release screening of all pharmaceutical advertising to ensure clarity and truthfulness. It furthermore suggests that physicians and pharmaceutical companies work jointly to create consumer advertising. It believes that the following statement should be a mandatory part of any consumer advertising for prescription drugs: "This medication is not appropriate for everyone. Consult your doctor about its appropriateness for you" (5).

Physician Considerations

The Case History presents a situation in which consumer advertising indirectly results in pressure on the physician. As the case also demonstrates, consumer advertising can play a positive role in alerting consumers to medical procedures or drugs with which they might not be familiar. Ultimately, however, a physician must intervene to determine whether the medical procedure and/or drug is appropriate for the patient.

The fact that Mr. Suit has predetermined which medication he should take before a diagnosis has been made will undoubtedly make the physician's job more difficult. But instead of becoming frustrated or discouraged, physicians should use this type of opportunity to educate patients and further develop the patient-doctor relationship. Given the time pressures in today's practice, figuring out how to do so will be a challenge.

Physicians have a duty, both individually and collectively, to advocate that everyone in the health care community adhere to the principles of beneficence and respect for autonomy. Physicians need to keep informed about consumer advertising so they can counsel patients knowledgeably and effectively, improve patient-physician communication, and enhance informed consent by patients. Physicians should also plan work-ups carefully, discuss them openly, and avoid unnecessary medications (4).

Physicians must refuse to compromise their medical judgment in the face of commercially induced pressures and educate their patients while remaining attentive to their concerns. Moreover, physicians individually and as a group can push for the creation of local, state, and national policies relating to consumer advertising, and they can monitor advertising and report inappropriate advertisements to relevant agencies such as the FDA. As individuals and as a profession, physicians must always be committed to the best interests of their patients and of society.

A similar version of this case study was originally published in ACP Observer in March 2000.

REFERENCES

1. USA Today. Americans pay more for medicine. 10 November 1999.
2. Kessler DA, Pines, WL. The federal regulation of prescription drug advertising and promotion. JAMA. 1990;264:2409-15.
3. Beauchamp TL, Childress JF. Principles of Biomedical Ethics, 4th ed. New York: Oxford University Press; 1994.
4. American College of Physicians. Ethics Manual, 4th ed. Ann Intern Med. 1998;128: 576-94.
5. Direct-to-Consumer Advertising for Prescription Drugs. ACP-ASIM position paper. October 1998 (www.acponline.org/hpp/pospaper/dtcads.htm).

ANNOTATED BIBLIOGRAPHY

American Medical Association. Current Opinions of the American Medical Association Council on Ethical and Judicial Affairs. Opinion 5.015. Direct-to-Consumer Advertisements of Prescription Drugs. June 1999.

Emphasizes the medical profession's need to ensure advertising guidelines are enforced and patient care is not compromised. Physicians should deny requests for inappropriate prescriptions and inform patients as to why certain drugs may not be suitable. At the same time, physicians should not be biased against drugs that are advertised.

Gemperli MP. MSJAMA: rethinking the role of the learned intermediary: the effect of direct-to-consumer advertising on litigation. JAMA. 2000;284:2241.

Discusses the "learned intermediary doctrine," which defines the legal boundaries of "failure to warn" suits formerly brought against pharmaceutical companies. However, the landmark case of Perez v. Wyeth Laboratories found the "learned intermediary doctrine" does not apply to direct-to-consumer advertising.

Hollon MF. Direct-to-consumer marketing of prescription drugs. JAMA. 1999;281:382-4.

Examines the profit motive behind direct-to-consumer marketing. Argues these advertisements provide little public health value and are more promotional material than educational information.

Holmer AF. Direct-to-consumer prescription drug advertising builds bridges between patients and physicians. JAMA. 1999;281:380-2.

A positive response to direct-to-consumer advertising by the President of the Pharmaceutical Research and Manufacturers of America. Seen as an excellent means of informing and empowering patients by communicating the availability of treatments to the public. States that this new empowerment of information does not conflict with physicians' prescribing authority.

Kravitz RL. MSJAMA: direct-to-consumer advertising of prescription drugs: implications for the patient-physician relationship. JAMA. 2000;284:2244.

Offers suggestions on how physicians can benefit from direct-to-consumer advertising. Physicians can direct patients' advertisement-prompted requests to a conversation about symptoms and concerns.

Murray E, Lo B, Pollack L, et al. Direct-to-consumer advertising: public perceptions of its effects on health behaviors, health care, and the doctor-patient relationship. J Am Board Fam Pract. 2004;17:6-18.

Direct-to-consumer advertising has positive and negative effects on health behaviors, health service utilization, and the patient-physician relationship. Effects are most prominent on individuals of low socioeconomic status. States that the benefits of encouraging hard-to-reach populations to seek preventive care must be balanced against increased health care costs resulting from clinically inappropriate requests generated by such advertising.

10

Documenting Sensitive Information: A Dilemma for Physicians

Commentary and Case History by Cynthia Clagett, MD,
Gail Povar, MD, and Karine Morin, LLM

Case History

Dr. Myra Ross, a general internist, works for Omnicare, a large managed care organization in the northwest United States. Omnicare provides health care on a contractual basis for the area's large military and civilian population.

Dr. Ross practices in one of Omnicare's primary care groups. She refers patients who need specialty care to several of the major medical centers in the community that have contracted with Omnicare. All medical records, including those of military personnel, are maintained in Omnicare's electronic database.

For the past 2 years Dr. Ross has been treating David Collins, a 39-year-old active-duty Army officer, for mild hyperlipidemia. David is an intelligence officer who plans to retire from the military in 3 years and work for the State Department. He is an engaging, quick-witted man whom Dr. Ross has come to know well. She looks forward to his visits as a break in her often monotonous clinical routine.

Today, as Dr. Ross enters the examining room, she notices that David is quiet and withdrawn. His posture is uncharacteristically slumped and his eyes, normally twinkling, are surrounded by darkened circles. He answers questions with monosyllabic responses and frequently asks Dr. Ross to repeat her questions.

Dr. Ross comments on David's unusual demeanor and asks if there is anything he would like to discuss. At first he stumbles, but soon reveals that a loved one has recently died. Upon further inquiry, David confesses that the loved one was his male companion of the past 12 years.

continued on page 64

Case History *continued from page 63*

His companion died in an auto accident 4 months ago. David feels he must remain silent to his supervisors about his loss. David tells Dr. Ross that if he disclosed his situation to his supervisor, he could forfeit his current position (and perhaps his pension) and would almost surely jeopardize future employment at the State Department. In fact, he has spoken to no one about this loss.

He expresses relief that he can finally unburden himself to Dr. Ross because she is a civilian physician. He explains that he has experienced changes in his weight and appetite, felt excessive guilt, and experienced intrusive passive suicidal ideation.

Dr. Ross diagnoses a major depressive disorder and feels that David would most benefit from both antidepressant medication and psychotherapy. David, however, flatly refuses the latter. "Doctor," he says, "there is no way my command wouldn't find out that I'm seeing a shrink. It would destroy my career. It's all I have left."

Dr. Ross tries to assure David that the medical record is confidential and that his supervisors are not routinely entitled to information in it. David shakes his head sadly and lets out a sigh. "Doctor, I can't believe you are so naive," he says. "I'm in Army intelligence. I can promise you there are 10 ways I could breach the confidentiality of the medical record system right now if I wanted."

Although David agrees to try an antidepressant and to see Dr. Ross more frequently, he asks her to refrain from writing anything about the depression in his chart. He also asks her to write his prescription on a paper pad and not enter it into the computer system as she ordinarily would do. Finally, David says he will pay for the medication himself rather than risk having a record of it in the Omnicare's prescription benefit database.

Dr. Ross knows she has an obligation to protect David's sensitive personal and medical information. She believes wholeheartedly that medical records should be kept confidential. However, she also believes David is justified in his skepticism about how well confidentiality is safeguarded. Nevertheless, she is uncomfortable prescribing a psychotropic medication without at least some note of it in the record. On the other hand, she fears that David will object to the treatment if she insists on any documentation. Untreated, he could very easily become much more depressed, even suicidal.

How should Dr. Ross proceed? Does she have an obligation to record the content and clinical plan of this clinic visit?

Commentary

The question posed in this case is whether physicians are required ethically and/or legally to record information that could, due to an increasingly accessible medical record, harm the well-being of patients. Inability to guarantee the confidentiality of sensitive and potentially harmful information strikes at the core requirement of the doctor-patient relationship: trust. Without trust, patients do not feel that they can disclose intimate and potentially embarrassing and/or damaging details of their lives that physicians need to diagnose and treat effectively.

Medical records are maintained primarily for the purpose of documenting and planning patient care (1). Increasingly, however, information contained in medical records serves other functions that range from review for reimbursement to quality care assessment. Records may also constitute a physician's strongest defense in the course of malpractice litigation (2). The content of records is dictated by these various purposes and also may be prescribed by statute. However, as a basic principle, the kind and amount of information included in a record should be determined by what is essential for patient care. Accurate and complete information is necessary to ensure that patients receive appropriate care.

The American College of Physicians Ethics Manual states that while the actual chart is the property of the physician or institution, the information contained in the chart is the property of the patient (3). The right of privacy, defined as the right of individuals to limit access by others to some aspect of one's person, includes information contained in medical records (4). Therefore "informational privacy" entails the right of an individual to control the dissemination and use of information that relates to himself or herself (5). Also, information disclosed in the course of a relationship between a patient and a physician is deemed confidential. This encourages patients to seek medical care and to discuss their problems candidly (3). The confidential nature of information shared in the course of physician-patient relationships is also meant to protect patients from harm that may result from information being used indiscriminately (5).

Medical confidentiality is not, however, absolute (3). Patients commonly sign waivers that authorize the disclosure of information in their medical records. More problematic, however, are instances where a physician may have a duty to disclose certain information without a patient's consent. Such a breach of confidentiality may be warranted only if the welfare of third parties outweighs the need to protect the privacy of the individual patient, as in the case of communicable diseases, child abuse, and knife or firearm wounds. Disclosure may also be required by law.

In this case, notations of a psychiatric illness carry the risk of potential discrimination that could destroy the patient's current and future employment if the information is insufficiently protected. Rules in the military or civilian government theoretically may prohibit superiors from accessing medical records without cause or from using psychiatric diagnoses in and of themselves as reasons to dismiss or deny promotion. Nevertheless, patients like David are justified in their concern that individual administrators may have significant latitude in how strictly such rules are interpreted and applied (6). Neither physicians nor patients can assume that rules regulating the use of patient information will effectively stop potential breaches of confidentiality.

Clinicians have additional ethical obligations, primary among them the imperative to "do no harm." An accurate medical record helps the health care team avoid unintended complications by alerting them to a patient's condition and current treatment. This is especially important during the inevitable episodes of cross-coverage. Significant depression such as David's is as potentially life threatening as many physical ailments; it must be detected and treated. Like other drugs, pharmacotherapies for depression carry the risk of significant side effects and may interact negatively with other medications. Failure to record significant diagnoses and therapies therefore puts patients at risk.

Because sensitive information regarding chronic medical problems can hurt an individual's ability to obtain insurance or even employment, the practice of keeping "double" records for patients like David has become more common. Alternatively, some clinicians within health care teams have created "code language" to obscure the true content of clinical interactions. Unfortunately, such practices beg the larger issue, which is the inability of electronic databases to protect the confidentiality of medical records.

Clearly, the advent of electronic charting (particularly within large integrated health care organizations), large databases, and computer prescription distribution has eroded the confidentiality of medical records. Already, the sale of data from these sources to insurers, private companies, government agencies, and financial institutions has become widespread, much in the same way as credit information is exchanged.

In theory, information that is protected by the doctor-patient privilege does not lose its confidentiality by being incorporated into a computer record (7). Additionally, the importance of confidentiality was extended by a recent Supreme Court decision that declared that the communication between a patient and a psychotherapist was privileged (8). Nevertheless, as David's own insight attests, no system of record keeping is completely immune to breaches of confidentiality. In fact, numerous lawsuits by HIV-infected patients and patients with other conditions have illustrated the legal consequences of unauthorized or illegitimate disclosure of information.

Legislation has been proposed to help protect the confidentiality of medical records in the computer age. One draft bill aims to establish uniform standards for handling medical records, to set procedures for obtaining consent for disclosure, and to define who can view records and under what circumstances. However, many commentators claim that the primary intent is to facilitate the computerization of records, which could lead to an even greater flow of information (9). The draft bill also includes several exceptions to the consent requirements and fails to address insider access to medical records, as in the case of staff members of a health care network or HMO. However, the legislation contains considerable penalties for infractions that may act as a deterrent. And although it is better known for making health insurance more portable, the Health Insurance Portability and Accountability Act, passed by Congress in August 1996, calls for security and confidentiality safeguards. Whether these will be sufficient in light of the increasing ability to exchange information remains questionable (10).

However, legal recourse for wrongful disclosure may be of little value to David. For example, he might be asked to authorize access to his medical record at the time of a promotion, placing him in a situation where he could hardly refuse to grant it. Thus, his fear relates not only to accessibility, but also to the very content of the record.

David seems to have accepted the need for some form of treatment and is willing to pay out-of-pocket, but he has genuine concerns about details of his condition being described in his chart. Dr. Ross must emphasize to David the benefits of a complete and accurate record. She should describe how another physician might need details of his care in order to avoid harming him, including emergencies in which David might not be physically able to provide such information himself. Dr. Ross should also explain Omnicare's mechanisms (if they exist) and legal requirements that limit access to sensitive information such as mental illness. She can inquire if there is an additional level of security to access such data, whether there is a record of who accesses the information, and if the system can identify attempts to violate access.

The 2-year relationship that evolved between Dr. Ross and David led him to reveal personal, intimate information that could jeopardize his employment if it were discovered by military personnel. Dr. Ross may wish to assure David that she will continue to hold his well-being and interest as paramount and emphasize that she wants to ensure he receives treatment for his depression. She can assure David that only essential data will be recorded. For instance, his homosexuality is not relevant to therapy for depression and need not be mentioned in this context; only his grief need be noted.

Furthermore, Dr. Ross should do all that she can to preserve the confidentiality of any information David provides. Finally, she should work with her colleagues to influence Omnicare's policies and contractual arrangements so that in the future she can help assure David and other patients that the confidentiality of their medical history is well protected by the systems to which they entrust their care.

A similar version of this case study was originally published in ACP Observer in December 1996.

REFERENCES

1. Bruce JAC. Privacy and Confidentiality of Health Care Information, 2nd ed. Chicago: American Hospital Publishing; 1988.
2. Privacy Protection Study Commission. Personal Privacy in an Information Society. Washington, DC: U.S. Government Printing Office; 1977.
3. American College of Physicians. Ethics Manual, 3rd ed. Ann Intern Med. 1992;117:947-60.
4. Gostin LO. Privacy and security of personal information in a new health care system. JAMA. 1993;270:2487-93.
5. Institute of Medicine. Health Data in the Information Age: Use, Disclosure and Privacy. Washington, DC: National Academy Press; 1994.
6. Howe E Jr. Uniformed Services University of Health Sciences; personal communication to Dr. G. Povar, June 18, 1996.
7. Cohen JD. HIV/AIDS confidentiality: are computerized medical records making confidentiality impossible? Software Law Journal. 1990;4:93-115.
8. Jaffee v. Redmond, No. 95-266, 1996 U.S. Lexis 3879 (US June 13, 1996).
9. Woodward B. Patients' Privacy at Risk. The New York Times. 15 November 1995.
10. Borzo G. Reform Law Boosts Electronic Records. American Medical News. 2 September 1996.

ANNOTATED BIBLIOGRAPHY

Annas, GJ. HIPAA regulations: a new era of medical record privacy? N Engl J Med. 2003;1486-90.

> *Provides a basic context for and summary of the first set of proposed regulations under the Health Insurance Portability and Accountability Act of 1996 (HIPAA). Notes that, whatever one's view of the HIPAA regulations, they will be the starting point for future national regulation of health care privacy.*

Bloche MG. Clinical loyalties and the social purposes of medicine. JAMA. 1999;281:268-74.

> *Discusses the dilemma that physicians face in the conflict between patient interests versus societal benefit.*

Department of Health and Human Services. Office for Civil Rights. Medical Privacy. National Standards to Protect the Privacy of Personal Health Information.

Health privacy resources, education materials, and FAQs on HIPAA privacy issues for consumers, health care providers, plans, and others from the Department of Health and Human Services. http://www.hhs.gov/ocr/hipaa/ (accessed May 25, 2004).

Jaffee v. Redmond, No. 95-266, 1996 U.S. Lexis 3879 (US June 13, 1996).

In general, legal matters require the gathering of all relevant evidence. However, some evidence is protected from disclosure in legal proceedings. Notably, this privilege is invoked to protect confidential communication between psychiatrists (or psychologists) and their clients. In the Jaffee decision, the Supreme Court held that such a privilege also applies to communications between licensed social workers and their clients in the course of psychotherapy.

11

The Older Impaired Driver

Commentary and Case History by Barbara Messinger-Rapport, MD,
Lois Snyder, JD, and Risa Lavizzo-Mourey, MD

Case History

Mr. Carr is a new patient. He is 85 years old, active, and lives alone in a small apartment in a suburb of Cleveland. He receives leupro-lide acetate (depot suspension) every 3 months for prostate cancer. He takes no other medication and has no other medical problems.

During a routine visit with Dr. Helms, memory problems surface in the conversation. Mr. Carr mentions that he got a little lost com-ing to the office, although it is less than a mile from home. On a mental state evaluation, he loses points for orientation, attention, calculation, recall, and visuospatial tasks. His total score is 18 out of 30. His blood pressure in the office is elevated at 180/85; his physical examination, however, including neuromuscular, vision, and fundu-scopic exams, is normal.

Dr. Helms recommends a driver's evaluation, but Mr. Carr refuses. "Why do that? What if the test doesn't turn out so well? I have to be able to get out of my apartment. I need to go to the grocery and drug store," he says.

Dr. Helms explains her concerns about Mr. Carr's ability to drive safely. Mr. Carr says he only drives during the day and always in his own neighborhood. He says he has no moving traffic violations. Still, Dr. Helms worries about Mr. Carr being injured or getting lost, and about his driving responsiveness, especially in poor weather. "I don't think I would want him to be out driving where my kids are walking home from school," she says to herself. But she is also concerned about restricting Mr. Carr's ability to get around and about patient confidentiality issues.

continued on page 71

Case History *continued from page 70*

It becomes difficult to continue a candid conversation. Dr. Helms makes a note to call Mr. Carr's son for more information after receiving Mr. Carr's permission to do so. In Ohio, there is no mandatory reporting law regarding drivers who are impaired by cognitive limitations. What else, if anything, should Dr. Helms do?

Commentary

Physicians may face several potential ethical conflicts when the issue of driver safety arises. The topic may surface where there is evidence of impaired cognition during an office visit or when a patient's family member approaches the physician to ask the physician to "order" a patient not to drive. Ethical issues of autonomy, beneficence, and nonmaleficence, as well as public health concerns, can be clearly identified in these scenarios. There are also implications for the physician's relationship with the patient and family.

Respect for the patient and for his decision to choose driving as a method of transportation and as a means of independence are important, as is patient confidentiality. Beneficence in certain settings may necessitate that physicians suggest altered driving patterns to improve driver safety because the oldest drivers have the highest per capita fatalities. Nonmaleficence suggests preventing the loss of independence, level of functioning, and possible depression that may ensue if driving is limited. Alternative transportation could even be dangerous if it requires waiting at secluded bus stops or crossing busy intersections. Physicians must balance the rights and privileges of individual patients with their responsibility to the community and the public health.

It is clear, however, that driving safety is within the purview of the physician. It is an instrumental activity of daily living, necessary for a person's independent functioning in the community. There is no single predictor of adverse driving events (moving violations, motor vehicle accidents) that can be applied in the office. Nevertheless, research suggests certain prognostic indicators. Therefore, health care providers must query, examine, and counsel their patients with respect to driving safety.

Background

As a group, older drivers are involved in motor vehicle accidents at a rate equal to or less than middle-aged drivers. However, the rate of older persons involved in fatal crashes rises after age 70. Compared with the fatality rate for drivers between the ages of 25 and 69, drivers 70 and over have a per mile fatality rate nine times as high. For drivers age 85 and over, the per mile fatality rate exceeds all groups, including that of teenagers (1).

The most common contributing factors in accidents and moving violations in older individuals include pulling out from the side of the road or changing lanes, careless backing, inaccurate turning, and difficulty giving right of way and reading traffic signs (2).

These accidents seldom involve high speeds or alcohol. Rather, problem driving in older adults involves visual, cognitive, and motor skills, which may decline with age. When compared with younger drivers, elderly individuals are more likely to be involved in accidents during the day, in good weather, at intersections, close to home, and involving two vehicles. In addition, they are more likely to be determined to be at fault by investigating officers (3).

The high fatality rate in the elderly population may be related to diminished physiological reserve. The higher mortality and morbidity with head trauma in the older patient may be explained by pre-existing central nervous system conditions such as degenerative brain disease or hydrocephalus, cerebrovascular disease, or central nervous system hypoperfusion. There is often concomitant chronic medical disease, including cardiovascular, pulmonary, and immunological disorders. Osteoporosis increases the risk of fracture. Corrected for severity of injury, elderly patients are five to six times more likely to die of similar injuries than younger drivers (3).

State Laws for Reporting Unsafe Drivers

State reporting laws vary regarding potentially unsafe drivers. Seven states (Pennsylvania, New Jersey, Delaware, Georgia, Nevada, Oregon, and California) require doctors to report health conditions that are hazardous to driving to licensing agencies. Some states require physicians to specify conditions such as epilepsy or dementia. All seven states give physicians who report unsafe drivers immunity from litigation. Ten states permit physician reporting, but Ohio and North Dakota do not grant immunity. Other jurisdictions permit physician reporting only after the patient has refused to report himself (4).

In states without immunity, physicians may be reluctant to report a potentially unsafe driver. Physicians should nonetheless report impaired drivers who clearly endanger themselves and/or the safety of the public and use their best judgment in determining when to report.

Physician-Patient Confidentiality

Confidentiality and respect for patient privacy are fundamental to medical care and the patient-physician relationship. Confidentiality, however, is not absolute and may have to be breached to protect individuals or the public, or to disclose information required by law. Before breaching confidentiality, physicians must ensure that they have made every effort to talk to patients about the issues. If confidentiality is to be breached, it should be done in a manner that minimizes harm to the patient (5).

Physician Obligation to the Potentially Unsafe Driver

Assessment of patient impairments that might result in unsafe driving is an ethical obligation. The goal of identifying the potentially unsafe older driver is to try to alter the driving behavior pattern before an adverse event occurs. Studies have not shown that chronic illness, functional status, or mental impairment consistently predict adverse events.

One recent study, however, demonstrated that the presence of heart disease, when adjusted for age, gender, and miles driven, predicted the adaptation of driving as well as the incidence of adverse driving events. It is not clear if it is the presence of heart disease or the side effect of the medications to treat the illness that is responsible for these predictions (6). Research has also shown that the inability to draw intersecting five-sided polygons was a better predictor than the Folstein Mini Mental Status Exam score or patients' recall ability, and this inability did identify those who quit vs. those currently driving.

There is even controversy about the safety of drivers who have been diagnosed with Alzheimer's disease. Post and Whitehouse suggest that persons diagnosed with probable Alzheimer's disease may be able to continue driving for 3 years after the initial diagnosis (7). Other experts feel that even early in the disease, there can be difficulty attending to multiple visual sources of input. Such a deficit in attending to and inhibiting appropriate stimuli could place even a mildly demented individual at risk as a driver (8).

Driver assessment courses have been developed to evaluate the visual and motor coordination and behind-the-wheel abilities of older persons. The most sophisticated courses are run by occupational therapists (OTs) who are certified in driver assessment and rehabilitation. These assessments are not designed to predict crash risk. Rather, they are designed to directly measure the effect of specific cognitive or physical deficits on driving skills. Many metropolitan areas have such programs.

Rehabilitation of the Older Driver

Typical recommendations of a licensed OT driver evaluation include 1) resume driving, 2) refrain from driving, 3) resume driving with vehicle adaptations, or

4) begin OT driver rehabilitation. Typically, OT driver rehabilitation for the elderly consists of 4 to 16 hours of treatment. This is a systematic program of therapy specifically designed to decrease a person's driving risk. It is only offered to those who demonstrate a good prognosis for resuming independent driving. Programs such as AARP's "55 Alive" also provide education programs for older drivers. (Some insurance companies discount policies for drivers who take such courses.)

The physician should consider counseling the partner of a slightly impaired older driver to continue or resume an equal share of the driving, with the patient's permission. Typically, married women do very little driving if the couple owns one car. However, it is important for married women to maintain their driving skills so they can maintain their independence if the husband's driving skills decline.

The physician must keep in mind that although these are reasonable recommendations, there are no hard data to show that these interventions will reduce future accidents.

Counseling the Potentially Unsafe Older Driver

Counseling a patient regarding driving behavior, even when the data are clear, can be difficult. Telling an older person to alter his driving habits and consider alternative forms of transportation can be devastating. It has been shown that people who relinquish their driving privileges suffer a sense of loss. It threatens self-esteem and personal dignity, and it implies social disability and dependency on others. Patients may deny the problem and resent what they see as physician intrusion.

Nonetheless, physicians must try to have an open conversation with their patients. The counseling process can be more effective and comfortable when the patient is prepared to deal with difficult news and when the physician provides information slowly, in small amounts, as if providing an abnormal biopsy report (9).

Once the patient is willing to consider a change in driving behavior, the physician may offer recommendations, which may include a referral to a licensed driver evaluation program. The physician should provide information about transportation alternatives. This information can be found at the Alzheimer's Association, the Office of the Aging, and the local Department of Transportation.

Conclusion

Dr. Helms needs to develop a continuing relationship with her patient, talk more with the patient and/or family, broaden her understanding about the nature and extent of the patient's cognitive and physical deficits, and help acquire information on transportation options that the patient may use if his driving ability is restricted in the future. Only then can she give her patient advice about driving.

Dr. Helms must balance the rights and privileges of her individual patient with her responsibility to the community and to the public health. If she determines that reporting is necessary because of a clear danger to the patient and/or the public, she must discuss this first with Mr. Carr. Even if it is too soon for that action, it is not too early to encourage Mr. Carr to think about how he will function without driving when the time comes.

Acknowledgments. The authors would like to thank Harvey L. Sterns, PhD, Professor of Psychology, University of Akron; and Ronni S. Sterns, PhD, Adjunct Fellow, Institute for Life-Span Development and Gerontology, University of Akron.

A similar version of this case study was originally published in ACP Observer in April 2000.

REFERENCES

1. U.S. Department of Transportation, National Highway Traffic Safety Administration, Traffic Safety Facts. DOT HS 808 955; 1998.
2. Assessing the Driving Ability of the Elderly: A Preliminary Investigation. Taira ED, ed. New York: Haworth Press; 1989.
3. Mandavia D, Newton K. Geriatric trauma. Emerg Med Clin North Am. 1998; 16:257-74.
4. U.S. Department of Transportation, National Highway Traffic Safety Administration, Safe Mobility for Older People Notebook. DOT HS 808 853; April 1999.
5. American College of Physicians. Ethics Manual, 4th ed. Ann Intern Med. 1998; 128:576-94.
6. Gallo JJ, Rebok GW, Lesikar SE. The driving habits of adults aged 60 years and older. J Am Geriatr Soc. 1999;47:335-41.
7. Post SG, Whitehouse PJ. Fairhill guidelines on ethics of the care of people with Alzheimer's disease: a clinical summary. Center for Biomedical Ethics, Case Western Reserve University and the Alzheimer's Association. J Am Geriatr Soc. 1995;43: 1423-9.
8. Duchek JM, et al. The role of selective attention in driving and dementia of the Alzheimer type. Alzheimer Dis Assoc Disord. 1997;11(Suppl 1):48-56.
9. Faulkner A, Maguire P, Regnard C. Breaking bad news: a flow diagram. Palliat Med. 1994;8:145-51.

Annotated Bibliography

Current Opinions of the American Medical Association Council on Ethical and Judicial Affairs. Opinion 2.24 Impaired Drivers and their Physicians. June 2000.

Discusses the responsibility of physicians to report patient driving impairments to state Departments of Motor Vehicles and the steps in this process.

Messinger-Rapport BJ, Rader E. High risk on the highway: how to identify and treat the impaired older driver. Geriatrics. 2000;55:32-4, 37-8, 41-2.

Finds that physicians and other health care providers may not be prepared to evaluate and advise the older patient on driving issues. Proposes two models to assist the clinician and patient through the process of restricting or curtailing driving by the older impaired patient.

12

Referrals and Patient Wishes
Commentary and Case History by Lois Snyder, JD

Case History

Internist Linda Curtis has been caring for Jack Green, age 48, and his wife, Betty, for 2 years, since the retirement of her partner, Dr. Smith. The Greens were Dr. Smith's patients for 18 years. Mr. Green is a small-business owner. He has never been seriously ill but is seeing his wife through a long illness with cancer. He seems depressed at a routine cholesterol check but, despite Dr. Curtis' attempts, is unwilling to talk. He does say that he hasn't felt like himself lately and complains of headaches, allergies, knee pain from an old jogging injury, and a rash on his face and elbows. "I need to feel better quick," he says, "I'd like to see a neurologist, orthopedic surgeon, and dermatologist. Who do you recommend?"

"Slow down," responds Dr. Curtis. "Let's see if I can't help you first." Mr. Green gets upset. "I really want these problems resolved now. I can't afford to feel under the weather, what with Betty sick. And I haven't been able to run very far lately." Running is Mr. Green's passion, and his primary exercise and stress relief.

After the examination, Dr. Curtis concludes that Mr. Green's problems do not warrant specialist intervention, not yet at least. She wonders how much of this is related to the pressure Mr. Green is under and the physical demands of caring for his wife. She tries again to get him to talk, without success.

"OK. I'd like to start you on steroid cream for your psoriasis and an antihistamine for your allergies. The headaches are likely related to the allergies and to stress. Your joint is stable, but I will talk to an orthopedic surgeon and determine whether a consultation is warranted. Let's see how it goes. I'd like you to come back next week."

continued on page 78

Case History *continued from page 77*

Dr. Curtis isn't convinced of the need for an orthopedist but feels pressured by Mr. Green's requests.

Dr. Curtis wants to talk further, but the patient cuts her off. "If you won't get me the help I need, I'll have to get it myself." An unhappy Mr. Green leaves, but he does take his prescription and schedules a follow-up appointment.

Dr. Curtis consults with an orthopedic surgeon, Sam Jackson, who, after hearing the history and evaluation, concurs that Dr. Curtis is on the appropriate course. Dr. Curtis makes a note to herself to check Mr. Green's insurance coverage. She has just started participating in HealthE, an IPA-model HMO, and she is learning its procedures. If Mr. Green is with HealthE, he will need written referrals to specialists for that care to be covered.

Mr. Green returns for his follow-up visit. His symptoms are beginning to improve but not enough to satisfy him. On further discussion he agrees that he doesn't really need to see a neurologist or dermatologist, but he remains emphatic about wanting to see an orthopedist. "Where's Dr. Smith when I need him? He would have recommended specialists to me at the last visit," says Mr. Green.

It turns out Mr. Green is a fee-for-service patient, so no written referral is needed. But he mentions that as part of the yearly review of benefits at his company, he is considering switching coverage for his family and his employees to an HMO, perhaps HealthE. "Would you be referring me if I had different coverage?" he asks. He says he is going to call his insurer to complain. How should Dr. Curtis handle this?

Commentary

When is a consultation warranted? The third edition of the American College of Physicians Ethics Manual states, "Physicians should obtain consultation when they feel a need for assistance in caring for the patient or when it is requested by the patient . . ." (1). Does this mean referrals should be made on demand? The short answer is, no.

Referrals should be made when they are in the patient's best interest. Determining what is in the patient's best interest is a matter of professional judgment and medical indication. This applies regardless of patient, peer, or institutional pressures about the cost of care, what type of insurance the patient has, or the physician's payment arrangement. However, with an insistent patient, this might be easier said than done.

"The welfare of the patient is always paramount in the consultation process," as it is in all aspects of the patient-physician relationship, states the Ethics Manual (1). The conflict here is in who is defining that welfare and how: the patient wants immediate intervention for what he sees as a problem requiring a specialist, whereas Dr. Curtis believes the issue for now is evaluation, which she is competent to handle. However, it is the physician who is in a better position to determine what is medically indicated. This is the basis of managed care policies placing the primary care physician in the role of "gatekeeper," even though it may limit the patient's freedom of choice.

Indeed, all physicians have an obligation to use health resources appropriately and efficiently, avoiding unnecessary tests (including unjustified repetition of tests) and unnecessary consultations. First and foremost, the physician must be a patient advocate. But being a patient advocate does not necessarily mean doing everything the patient wants. And the traditional approach to patient advocacy is also being challenged by the need to be conscious of societal and institutional concerns about resource allocation (2).

Here Dr. Curtis sees no societal or institutional-patient conflict. She believes, and the orthopedic surgeon concurs, that she is on the right course in evaluating and following Mr. Green's knee condition. Dr. Curtis' greatest challenge is effectively communicating this to Mr. Green. Physician and patient must thoroughly discuss their concerns and expectations. Dr. Curtis may not be able to change Mr. Green's expectations (although she was successful regarding the dermatologist and neurologist), but she is right to try. She should continue to do so by informing the patient about her approach to care, the need to allow time for healing, and her discussion with Dr. Jackson.

Physicians should try to help patients develop realistic expectations about medical care. More care is not always better care, and tests carry risk and can result in false positives, increasing stress and leading to potential complications. Perhaps for the patient's previous physician, Dr. Smith, being a patient advocate meant doing what the patient wanted and doing more, although nearly 20 years ago there was less "more" to do.

The Greens are fee-for-service patients, which Dr. Curtis did not know at the time of her original recommendation. The payment arrangement was, correctly, not part of her thinking about a care plan for Mr. Green. Payment arrangements could be a subtle, or not so subtle, influence on clinical judgment. An HMO doctor could take a wait-and-see approach for too long. Under some contractual arrangements with HMOs, for example, physicians agree to a percentage withholding of their fees that is returned only if their referral account for specialist and laboratory services has a surplus at the end of the year. Often there are also bonuses for running a surplus. In the fee-for-service context, a physician could too quickly order, or repeat, a test or make a referral because of the financial incentive to do more and therefore be paid more (2,3).

Mr. Green has said he is considering changing coverage. Under the rules of HealthE, patients need a written referral from the primary care physician for care by a specialist to be covered. Dr. Curtis needs to discuss this with the patient, and encourage him to talk to HealthE about the details of coverage, so that he understands the rationale behind pre-authorized referrals and other terms of coverage. Such an understanding is essential if Mr. Green is to make an informed choice among insurance plans.

Mr. Green has also said that he will complain to his current insurer, which he is free to do. He may even start to talk about legal action. But the practice and documentation of medically appropriate care are the best defenses to challenges regarding that care, legal or otherwise.

If after several weeks of conservative management Mr. Green is not better, or if there is evidence of a ligament injury or increased swelling, Dr. Curtis will want to rethink her position on referral. But for now, referral seems unnecessary and not beneficial to the patient.

It is likely that if Mr. Green remains adamant about seeing an orthopedist now, he will find one on his own. If on a subsequent visit Mr. Green persists in wanting names, Dr. Curtis should at that point give him some names of physicians she usually recommends. If he switches to HealthE, she should explain to Mr. Green that physician visits, tests, and treatment without a referral would be at the patient's expense. Regardless of the insurance coverage, Dr. Curtis should indicate that she believes this is not medically indicated nor in Mr. Green's best interest at this time.

A similar version of this case study was originally published in ACP Observer in March 1995.

REFERENCES

1. American College of Physicians. Ethics Manual, 3rd ed. Ann Intern Med. 1992; 117:947-60.
2. Wolf SM. Health care reform and the future of physician ethics. Hastings Center Report. 1994;24:28-41.
3. Hillman AL. Health maintenance organizations, financial incentives and physicians' judgments. Ann Intern Med. 1990;112:891-3.
4. Rodwin MA. Medicine, Money, and Morals: Physicians' Conflicts of Interest. New York: Oxford University Press; 1993.

ANNOTATED BIBLIOGRAPHY

Miles SH. Informed demand for "non-beneficial" medical treatment. N Engl J Med. 1991;325:512-5.

The context here is the Helga Wanglie case and a family's fight to continue life-sustaining treatment against medical advice. But the argument is applicable: patient desires do not create an entitlement to inappropriate care.

Wolf SM. Health care reform and the future of physician ethics. Hastings Center Report. 1994;24:28-41.

Discusses ethical tensions inherent in various health care delivery models and in efforts at cost consciousness and containment; analyzes proposals for clarifying physician obligations and proposes the development of a new ethics of institutions.

13

Patient Prejudice

Commentary and Case History by Errol D. Crook, MD, and Lois Snyder, JD

Case History

Mr. Smith is a 60-year-old white male who presents to his internist, Dr. Johnson, complaining of intermittent chest pain for several days. Dr. Johnson has cared for Mr. Smith for many years and knows that he would not complain about anything unless he was having significant problems. His pain is occurring at lower and lower levels of physical activity and sometimes when he is resting. After examining Mr. Smith and performing an EKG, Dr. Johnson is concerned about the possibility of unstable angina and decides that Mr. Smith needs to be admitted to the hospital for further evaluation and treatment.

Dr. Johnson admits Mr. Smith to the intensive care unit. He asks Dr. Natal, a Board-certified cardiologist, to see Mr. Smith. Dr. Johnson and his partner have referred many of their cardiac patients to Dr. Natal for several years, believing him to be quite thorough and very good with patients. All of their patients have seemed happy with Dr. Natal's care.

Dr. Natal sees Mr. Smith that afternoon. As the doctor is taking his history, Mr. Smith starts to experience typical anginal chest pain associated with some mild EKG changes. Dr. Natal is able to relieve his pain with sublingual nitroglycerin and intravenous anti-anginal agents, but he feels that cardiac catheterization is warranted. He discusses the events with Mr. Smith and makes plans to perform the procedure in the morning. Mr. Smith is hesitant but agrees to have the procedure if Dr. Johnson is in favor. The patient has two more episodes of chest pain that afternoon.

Dr. Johnson comes by later, after having discussed Mr. Smith's care with Dr. Natal. He tells Mr. Smith that he agrees the catheterization is

continued on page 83

> **Case History** *continued from page 82*
>
> needed. Mr. Smith responds, "I know that I need something done, but will you be there?" As Dr. Johnson is explaining that he will not be present during the procedure, he senses that Mr. Smith is becoming upset. He asks what is wrong.
>
> "Dr. Johnson," Mr. Smith starts hesitantly, "I would rather have another cardiologist." Dr. Johnson replies that Dr. Natal is very good and sees a lot of his patients. Mr. Smith is still not satisfied. After further discussion that includes questions about Dr. Natal's medical training and heritage, it becomes obvious that Mr. Smith is not comfortable with a "foreign doctor."
>
> Dr. Johnson is quite surprised. With respect, he attempts to convince the patient that Dr. Natal has his full support and utmost confidence. He reiterates, "Dr. Natal is very well-trained and is one of the most respected cardiologists in the area." Mr. Smith remains steadfast in his desire for another cardiologist.
>
> What should Dr. Johnson do? Should he continue in his efforts to convince Mr. Smith of Dr. Natal's qualifications? Should he inform Dr. Natal that Mr. Smith wants a different doctor? Should he suggest that Mr. Smith tell Dr. Natal himself?

Commentary

Establishing a good patient-physician relationship is primary to the practice of medicine. Maintaining that marriage between physician and patient often requires handling quite delicate and complex issues. No longer is this relationship paternalistic, with the physician acting as the sole decision-maker; instead, it is a partnership with shared decision-making. Differences in culture, religion or certain, ideological beliefs may strain and, in some cases, sever the union. This case demonstrates how perceived differences can threaten a patient-physician relationship and affect patient care.

Discrimination of any kind toward patients or colleagues has no place in medicine. A physician may not discriminate against a class or category of patients (1). Patients are obviously not bound by a professional code of conduct, as are physicians, although one would hope that they would not practice or tolerate discrimination. Patients have their own aims and values, which play a major role in their care.

Dr. Johnson is faced with a serious dilemma. What he believes is best for the patient, best for a peer, and consonant with his ideas of right and wrong appear to be a potential threat to his patient's confidence in him. And, as the American College of Physicians Ethics Manual states, "The patient's welfare and best interests must be the physician's main concern . . . In all instances, the physician must help maintain the dignity of the person and respect the uniqueness of each person" (1). Dr. Johnson's actions must be guided by these principles.

His primary concern has to be for Mr. Smith, his patient of many years. Dr. Johnson has his patient's best interest in mind by referring to Dr. Natal. This must be communicated, and it is reasonable for Dr. Johnson to attempt to convince Mr. Smith of Dr. Natal's medical expertise. It is also imperative that Dr. Johnson keep Mr. Smith well-informed about the consequences of his decision. If, for instance, Dr. Natal were the only cardiologist in the area, Mr. Smith would have to transfer to another facility to avoid being under Dr. Natal's care. However, this must be done in a gentle, non-offensive manner that respects Mr. Smith's uniqueness (3).

The reasons for Mr. Smith's request should be examined. It may be uncomfortable for Dr. Johnson to have to elicit from the patient what the problem is here, but he needs to do so both to resolve this situation and to inform his decisions about subsequent referrals. When female patients request female physicians, many physicians will try to comply without question. Sometimes a patient will request a physician with whom he has had a prior relationship, or one who was recommended by a family member, or an older, "more experienced" doctor. In other circumstances, there could be communication barriers that interfere with the provision of care. But here, there are no language problems. And although physician communication styles and personalities can result in different comfort levels for patients, Dr. Johnson knows Dr. Natal to have generally good communication skills and a good bedside manner.

The distinction between patient preferences and discrimination can sometimes be cloudy, although not in this case. Mr. Smith's request is based on his biases against people who do not share his cultural background. This should be challenged, but without undermining the patient's condition or the patient-physician relationship. Although the reasons that Mr. Smith has asked for another cardiologist may seem unreasonable, it is his prerogative to do so. Dr. Johnson is correct to try to educate him, but, ultimately, he does not need to agree with or understand Mr. Smith's wishes. Those wishes must be respected, however, because the patient has the right to choose. Dr. Johnson must recognize that each patient comes into the relationship with his or her own set of values and desires. If Dr. Johnson believes that Dr. Natal is being unfairly discriminated against and does not want to be in any way involved, he has the option of recommending a physician to take his place and withdrawing from the case.

Clearly, physicians aren't immune from biases against certain groups. The same biases in American culture are found in American medicine. Such discrimination persists despite laws that prohibit it in many areas of public life. A physician like Dr. Natal may experience even more discrimination because of an "unusual" name, a particular complexion, a different manner of dress or an accent. Many international medical graduates have suffered from discrimination. They could experience bias from patients, and from hospitals, training programs, and other physicians as well (3). Where medical training occurs is not the only determinant: U.S.-trained physicians of foreign birth or ancestry have experienced the same problems. They often find it difficult to get referrals and in some cases to get privileges.

What should Dr. Johnson do to keep his professional relationship with Dr. Natal a strong one? Although Dr. Johnson's primary obligation is to his patient, he also has a professional obligation to his colleague. He must not allow this episode or the chance that similar occurrences may happen to sway his referral pattern. There is no question of Dr. Natal's qualifications and abilities as a physician, and past referrals have had excellent results.

It would not be appropriate, and might damage his relationship with the patient, for Dr. Johnson to insist that Mr. Smith tell Dr. Natal about his wishes himself. Does Dr. Johnson have an obligation to inform Dr. Natal about all of this? Physicians should treat not only their patients, but also each other, with respect. Dr. Johnson should assure Dr. Natal that he has his continued support and confidence and that this incident will not change his referral practices in any way.

Because the United States is made up of diverse peoples that sometimes clash, it is important to learn and exercise the skills to solve problems when they arise, and to help patients to learn. Many physicians may face problems similar to those faced by Dr. Johnson. As professionals, physicians occupy positions of significant influence. Therefore, they can, and should, move communities away from bigotry, not just by their words but by their actions.

A similar version of this case study was originally published in ACP Observer in December 1994.

REFERENCES

1. American College of Physicians. Ethics Manual, 3rd ed. Ann Intern Med. 1992;117: 947-60.
2. Brock DW, Wartman SA. When competent patients make irrational choices. N Engl J Med. 1990;322:1595-9.
3. Doyle E. Foreign-born doctors charge discrimination, fight back with grievances, court challenges. ACP Observer. December 1993; Vol. 13, No. 11.

ANNOTATED BIBLIOGRAPHY

Brock DW, Wartman SA. When competent patients make irrational choices. N Engl J Med. 1990;322:1595-9.

Patients have a right to make unusual treatment decisions if they are competent. Physicians, however, may try to convince patients to reconsider irrational choices. This article distinguishes unusual treatment decisions from irrational choices and discusses physician and patient roles in shared treatment decision-making.

14

Do You Need to Tell Patients About Mistakes?

Commentary and Case History by Vincent E. Herrin, MD

Case History

Dr. Jinks was in a hurry. She'd had several calls that day and more than her average number of patients in the hospital. Then one of her newer patients, Mrs. Redd, asked for an antibiotic for her cough and fever. "I've had pneumonia before," Mrs. Redd reminded her.

After examining the patient, Dr. Jinks concluded that Mrs. Redd met the criteria for outpatient treatment of pneumonia. After she glanced at the outside of the chart and saw no allergy warning sticker, she asked the nurse to give Mrs. Redd ceftriaxone.

About 30 minutes later, the nurse rushed in and said that Mrs. Redd was having a "bad reaction." Dr. Jinks hurried to her patient and found her wheezing and covered with hives. Her blood pressure was also falling. Dr. Jinks acted quickly to treat her anaphylaxis, and in a short time Mrs. Redd was feeling much better. Her daughter thanked Dr. Jinks profusely and commented on how cool she had been under pressure. Mrs. Redd was also thankful, but a little frustrated. "I guess I'll never be able to take antibiotics," she sighed. "I can't believe I've had another reaction."

Dr. Jinks was taken aback. She asked Mrs. Redd to remain in the treatment room for observation and rushed back to her office. Glancing through the patient's chart, she found Mrs. Redd's history from her first visit. She had listed cephalexin under allergies, with a note explaining "bad rash." Somehow Dr. Jinks had missed the note and neglected to fill in the allergy box on the outside of the chart. Evidently the office staff had missed it too.

continued on page 88

> **Case History** *continued from page 87*
>
> Although Mrs. Redd had recovered quickly and was going to be fine, Dr. Jinks wondered what she should tell her patient about her error.
>
> Does Dr. Jinks need to mention the mistake? After all, the patient and her daughter might lose trust in her. No permanent physical harm had been done, but the disclosure could cause long-lasting emotional harm to their relationship.

Commentary

Although errors are inevitable in medical practice, physicians receive little guidance or training about what to do when they make a mistake. When should physicians tell patients about an error? Does it matter if no lasting harm has been done? Should physicians factor patient characteristics into the decision? Should public perception of the profession matter?

One leading medical ethics textbook claims that for thousands of years, physicians have generated their own codes of ethics with little or no input from society and little consideration for societal expectations. These codes "have rarely appealed . . . to a source of moral authority beyond the traditions and judgments of physicians" (1).

Still, one might argue that for the most part, society's expectations have rarely differed from the standards that physicians set for themselves. Over the past couple of generations, however, these expectations have changed profoundly, due in large part to the patients' rights movement that began in the 1960s.

Until 1980, the American Medical Association's code of ethics offered little guidance about the obligation to disclose. Physicians were simply admonished to "deal honestly with patients and colleagues" (2).

Although the Ethics Manual of the American College of Physicians is more definitive, it still leaves room for individual physician judgment. It states: "Physicians should disclose to patients information about procedural or judgment errors made in the course of care if such information is material to the patient's well-being. Errors do not necessarily constitute improper, negligent, or unethical behavior, but failure to disclose them may" (3).

Public Perceptions

Although mistakes have long been part of everyday practice, news stories about the frequency of medical errors have received much more attention over the past decade. In particular, the number of errors cited in the Institute of Medicine report on patient safety alarmed the medical profession and the public (4).

The Institute of Medicine report spurred physicians and health care organizations to step up efforts to assess and reduce medical mistakes, but it left many in the general public thinking that the medical establishment is not trustworthy. Although the number of errors cited in the Institute of Medicine report has since been challenged, the public's wariness has been reinforced by repeated news reports that visiting a doctor's office or hospital may be hazardous to your health.

The public's mistrust of medicine was underscored by a recent newscast about a surgical error. The reporter noted that the story was shocking not because the error occurred but because the hospital actually admitted that its staff made a mistake.

Physicians have struggled with disclosure in part because they expect perfection from themselves and each other. As one physician-author commented, "Physicians, not unlike test pilots, come to view an error as a failure of character— you weren't careful enough, you didn't try hard enough" (5).

Such unrealistic expectations make it difficult to admit to a mistake. These expectations begin to arise very early in medical training. One study of interns and residents who had made medical mistakes found that young physicians disclosed only about one-quarter of their mistakes to the patient or family (6). If medical trainees are not learning to discuss errors, is there any chance they will become more forthcoming as they enter practice?

Culture of Silence

The medical profession is not entirely to blame for its "culture of silence." Patients have high expectations for their practitioners. As one commentator remarked: "Perhaps the only people who seem to demand perfection more than doctors are patients" (7). A physician wrote: "If the medical profession has no room for doctors' mistakes, neither does society" (8).

Doctors' and patients' unrealistic expectations reinforce each other. Patients and physicians alike expect perfection, and society demands full disclosure, yet any error is perceived as a character flaw and grounds for a lawsuit.

Most physicians and patients would likely agree that the patient-physician relationship is based on confidence and trust. Doctors expect their patients to tell them the truth about their medical histories and health behaviors that might affect their medical care. Patients expect their physicians to be competent, to respect privacy and confidentiality, and to be truthful.

But the fact remains that the relationship is an unequal one because physicians have the advantage of specific knowledge and experience. Physicians also usually know the results of labs, biopsies, radiographic studies, and other tests before their patients do, and they must assimilate and convey this information to their patients.

Patients are not powerless, however, and often have as much or more to do with the success or failure of the patient-physician relationship as the physician. A patient may choose to switch physicians or advise friends and neighbors to avoid a certain doctor. A patient may be dishonest about his or her medical and social history or refuse to follow medical advice or treatments. Additionally, the patient's power to sue looms over physician-patient disagreements, poor outcomes, and even simple mistakes.

Patient-Physician Relationship

In this case, Dr. Jinks wonders if she should tell the patient that a mistake was made because no lasting harm was done. There may be instances where revealing a mistake might only cause alarm. Dr. Jinks may feel that Mrs. Redd will lose trust in her if the truth is revealed. Mrs. Redd might even find another doctor.

Dr. Jinks may be tempted to selectively apply the dictum, "First, do no harm," reasoning that because the problem was easily resolved, telling the patient about the incident could damage their relationship. Moreover, she may have a legitimate desire to protect Mrs. Redd and her family from additional concern about their health care.

However, do patients want to be protected in this way? One study questioned patients about hypothetical error scenarios that were categorized as mild, moderate, and severe. Across the board, patients said they wanted physicians to acknowledge an error. In the case of severe errors, many patients reported that they might indeed switch physicians or file suit, even if the physician was honest. Patients, however, said they were even more inclined to drop or sue a physician who had not disclosed a severe error and they learned about it through other means (9).

Systemic Error

Because many physicians in today's practice environment work as employees or have contracts with health care organizations, admitting mistakes can be even more difficult. Health care organizations often pin blame for an error on an individual provider rather than attempting to make systemic changes to avoid similar problems in the future. Studies of other industries in which errors carry grave consequences (aviation is a prime example) have revealed that singling out individuals for shame and blame does not encourage honesty or correct ongoing problems (10).

Admissions of mistakes and investigations into errors should not end simply with an assignment of blame. Organizations and physicians should instead engage in an ongoing process to identify ways to improve care.

Last year, the Joint Commission on Accreditation of Healthcare Organizations (JCAHO) adopted new patient safety standards that may help develop a "culture of safety." As part of its accreditation process, JCAHO now requires health care organizations to disclose unanticipated injuries, investigate their root causes, and take action to prevent their recurrence. It is unclear how JCAHO may measure compliance with this new standard, but health care organizations will have to educate staff about this initiative to show JCAHO that they are taking appropriate steps.

Solutions

Dr. Jinks should not feel alone. Although they are common, mistakes put tremendous pressure on physicians as they struggle with which course to take and how to be "most ethical." Dr. Jinks is rightly concerned about her patient's potential negative response, and she wants to avoid adding uncertainty to the patient-physician relationship.

Although some physicians find that admitting a mistake is very therapeutic (11), Dr. Jinks considers keeping the situation to herself, not as a self-serving gesture but to avoid burdening the patient and family. But would silence be in the patient's best interests? What if Mrs. Redd finds out anyway or is too frightened to try another antibiotic the next time she needs one?

Dr. Jinks should give strong consideration to admitting her mistake honestly and apologetically. Mrs. Redd may gain a new sense of security with the knowledge that she has an honest, caring physician. If the relationship with this patient is shattered by this admission and the patient seeks care elsewhere, Dr. Jinks might be better off knowing this now.

Finally, Dr. Jinks should not pass up the opportunity to evaluate and improve her practice procedures. She should review what happened in this case with her office staff rather than attempt to assign blame to someone else for the missing allergy sticker. Indeed, if physicians incorporated regular evaluation and improvement efforts into their routines, many medical errors could be avoided. Still, we cannot correct the process without also convincing physicians to openly acknowledge their mistakes.

The American public can be judgmental, and it tends to lose faith in institutions when flaws are revealed. There is no reason, however, that the medical profession has to suffer that fate. Considering medicine's unique relationship with society, we can improve our profession only through honesty, forthrightness, and a willingness to address flaws in our systems. Improvement has to start with physicians, and Dr. Jinks is in a good position to do something important. Society wants the truth, and there is rarely a good reason to hide it.

A similar version of this case study was originally published in ACP Observer in March 2002.

REFERENCES

1. Beauchamp TL, Childress JF. Principles of Biomedical Ethics, 5th ed. Oxford: University Press; 2001:7.
2. American Medical Association. Current Opinions of the Council on Ethical and Judicial Affairs of the American Medical Association. Chicago: American Medical Association; 1981:ix.
3. American College of Physicians. Ethics Manual, 4th ed. Ann Intern Med. 1998; 128:576-94.
4. Institute of Medicine. To Err Is Human: Building a Safer Health System. Washington, DC: National Academy Press; 1999.
5. Leape LL. Error in medicine. JAMA. 1994;272:1851-7.
6. Wu AW, Folkman S, McPhee S, Lo B. Do house officers learn from their mistakes? JAMA. 1991;265:2089-94.
7. Snyder L, Brennan TA. Disclosure of errors and the threat of malpractice. In: Snyder L, ed. Ethical Choices: Case Studies for Medical Practice. Philadelphia: American College of Physicians; 1996:49.
8. Hilfiker D. Healing the Wounds. New York: Pantheon Books; 1985.
9. Witman AB, Park DM, Hardin SB. How do patients want physicians to handle mistakes? Arch Intern Med. 1996;156:2565-9.
10. Berwick DM, Leape LL. Reducing errors in medicine. BMJ. 1999;319:136-7.
11. Howe EG. Possible mistakes. J Clin Ethics. 1997;8:323-8.

ANNOTATED BIBLIOGRAPHY

Calman NS. No one needs to know. Health Affairs. 2001;20:243-9.

> *A doctor recalls his own painful involvement in a medical error cover-up. He advocates that doctors admit and openly discuss mistakes to improve care.*

Finkelstein D, Wu AW, Holtzman NA, Smith MK. When a physician harms a patient by a medical error: ethical, legal, and risk management considerations. J Clin Ethics. 1997;8:330-5.

> *Although a physician's legal and risk management responsibilities may conflict with the ethical responsibility of disclosure of a medical error, disclosure is the most appropriate way to show respect and establish mutual trust in patient-physician relationships.*

Leape LL. Error in medicine. JAMA. 1994;272:1851-7.

Examines the potential for error in medicine, attitudes toward errors and prevention, and possible systems changes to prevent or identify errors in a timely fashion.

Mazor KM, Simon SR, Yood RA, et al. Health plan members' views about disclosure of medical errors. Ann Intern Med. 2004;140:409-18.

Found that patients are likely to respond more favorably to physicians who fully disclose medical errors than to physicians who are less forthright, but case facts and the severity of the clinical outcome also affect how patients respond.

Rosner F, Berger JT, Kark P, et al. Disclosure and prevention of medical errors (Committee on Bioethical Issues of the Medical Society of the State of New York). Arch Intern Med. 2000;160:2089-92.

A comprehensive discussion of medical errors that includes a definition of error, examination of medical society guidelines, discussion of disclosure, and systems and other major issues. Finds honest, full disclosure to be a duty of the physician when an error has occurred.

15

Disclosure of Errors and the Threat of Malpractice

Commentary by Lois Snyder, JD, and Troyen A. Brennan, MD, JD, MPH
Case History by Troyen A. Brennan, MD, JD, MPH

Case History

Dr. Howard McGregor has been concerned about his busy internal medicine practice. He has contracts with several managed care plans and is now seeing an average of 16 patients per half-day session. As little as 3 years ago, he was seeing only nine patients per session. Sometimes he wonders if he is adequately following up on tests and procedures.

Today he is seeing Karen Madner, a 53-year-old woman whom he has followed since she was in her late 30's. She has had three children and a subsequent tubal ligation. She is very concerned about breast cancer because her mother and sister both died from it after having received a late diagnosis. They died at ages 48 and 40, respectively. She no longer sees an obstetrician/gynecologist; Dr. McGregor provides her gynecological care.

It has been approximately 16 months since Ms. Madner's last visit. She usually has a yearly follow-up, at which time she receives a pap smear and a mammogram. In reviewing the record before Ms. Madner comes in, Dr. McGregor is shocked to find that the previous mammogram report (16 months before) had suggested an abnormality and called for follow-up in 4 months. The radiologist's note was fairly explicit about the suspicious nature of this lesion and the need for expedient follow-up. Dr. McGregor has no idea how he could have overlooked this report.

He examines Ms. Madner and finds a palpable lump in the area

continued on page 95

94

Case History *continued from page 94*

of the abnormality. At this point he is very anxious and irritated. He questions Ms. Madner about her use of breast self-examination, which she says she does religiously, and suggests that she needs a mammogram immediately and also should be referred to a breast surgeon. "What's going on?" she asks. "I had a normal mammogram last time." Ms. Madner is, of course, quite upset as well, but Dr. McGregor is so agitated he does a poor job of attending to her emotional concerns.

After Ms. Madner leaves, Dr. McGregor has some time for reflection. He recalls that Ms. Madner is a single mother who works full-time to support her two high-school-aged children. The treatment for breast cancer could have significant impact on her ability to continue to work. He wonders if she has disability insurance and makes a note to ask her.

Dr. McGregor then calls his senior colleague, Dr. Rendler, for advice. Dr. Rendler is surprised that Dr. McGregor did not have a more engaging discussion with the patient. Dr. Rendler believes that full disclosure of mistakes with patients is the best course. She explains that she has had similar cases in the past and has found that the outcome has always been best when one honestly shares one's mistakes with the patient. Patients are less likely to sue if so informed and are better able to cope with the disease.

Dr. McGregor considers what to do next. What should he decide?

Commentary

To err is human. No one is immune. But when physicians err, the stakes obviously can be quite high.

The issue here is not how to eliminate error, an unobtainable goal. Nonetheless, it clearly influences the culture and world view of medicine. One physician's view of mistakes: "It is a crime . . . There's some anonymous court that's been set up someplace—I mean Osler or God somewhere at Massachusetts General Hospital—and you've been convicted and tried at the same time" (1).

Physicians, perhaps by nature and certainly as a result of their education and training, often strive to attain perfection in the practice of medicine (2,3). Commenting on this phenomenon, Lucian Leape has observed: "One result is that physicians, not unlike test pilots, come to view an error as a failure of character—you weren't careful enough, you didn't try hard enough" (3). This sensibility often becomes very pronounced among residents (see Chapter 25).

Patients are perhaps the only people who seem to demand perfection in medicine more than doctors. They sometimes have unrealistic expectations about what medicine, and their physicians, can do for them, and about the possibility of error in the provision of health care. This, too, influences how physicians handle mistakes. Physicians should keep patients well-informed and help them to have reasonable expectations. Patients, however, should reasonably expect that their physicians will give their care appropriate attention and follow-up. It is the physician's obligation to do so.

Of course, errors should be prevented when possible. But some number of mistakes are inevitable, sometimes due to negligence, sometimes not. And the potential for errors is great in a complicated endeavor like medicine and in complex settings such as hospitals. The Harvard Study of New York hospitals found that among discharges from a random sample of 51 hospitals, 1% of patients suffered harm as the result of negligence (4). In another study, intensive care unit patients were found to have been subject to an average of 178 separate "activities" per day each and 1.7 errors per day each, 29% of which could be characterized as potentially serious or fatal (3).

Reflecting on this study, Dr. Leape notes that 1.7 errors per day means a 99% proficiency rate. But, he finds, 1% error is much greater than that found acceptable in, for example, dangerous industries such as aviation and nuclear power. He concludes that although physicians, nurses, and pharmacists "probably are among the most careful professionals in our society," they are not proficient at error prevention because "they have a great deal of difficulty in dealing with human error when it does occur" (3). It also may not be immediately apparent who was responsible for the mistake, or individuals may deny responsibility (5).

Which brings us to the issue at hand: how to deal with error while maintaining ethical obligations to the patient and respecting patient rights.

The third edition of the American College of Physicians Ethics Manual directs physicians to "disclose to patients information about procedural or judgment errors made in the course of care, if such information significantly affects the care of the patient" (6). It goes on to say that "Errors do not necessarily constitute improper, negligent, or unethical behavior" (6). But failure to disclose a significant error can be all three.

It is necessary and important for Dr. McGregor to have a longer discussion with Ms. Madner about the previously overlooked lesion on the mammogram. Ms. Madner has a right to information that significantly affects her care. She also needs to make further decisions about her care and to be well-informed in order to make those decisions and work in partnership with Dr. McGregor. "Effective patient-physician communication can dispel uncertainty and fear and enhance healing and patient satisfaction" (6). It can also help dispel the anger and confusion that often contribute to the filing of malpractice lawsuits.

The threat of legal action is a real one. Most liability insurers would likely want to be notified very early on, at the discovery of the mistake or shortly thereafter. Although the physician might hold himself or herself to a standard of perfection, however, the legal system does not. Instead, what is required is that the physician practice with reasonable care, that is, as a similarly trained physician would do in similar circumstances.

Apart from potentially preventing legal action, effective communication can help maintain or restore the trust necessary to a good patient-physician relationship. In this instance, Ms. Madner clearly knows or will know shortly that something went awry. This is not an error undetectable to the lay person. Even if it were, the standard for disclosure is not detectability. It is whether or not information about the error will significantly affect the patient's care. It is unethical to say nothing here, and that course of action would undermine or ultimately destroy the relationship.

Dr. McGregor is right to be very concerned about the potential consequences of the mistake and of disclosure, and to give thought to how he will broach the discussion with the patient and what he might say. He might further discuss this with Dr. Rendler, while maintaining patient confidentiality, in preparation for his conversation with Ms. Madner. He will also want to think about changes in his practice or office procedures that will help him avoid such mistakes in the future, for example, a review of his patient load and attention to how lab reports are screened. Acknowledging an error and accepting responsibility for it can be first steps in improvements in quality of care. He should, however, have his discussion with the patient sooner rather than later and her care should not be further delayed.

Dr. McGregor might also benefit from any support Dr. Rendler or another colleague can provide him. The emotional impact of the mistake process can take a toll on the physician. "The medical profession simply seems to have no place for its mistakes. There is no permission given to talk about errors, no way of venting emotional responses. Indeed, one would almost think that mistakes are in the same category as sins . . . " (2). Physicians should find a place to talk about mistakes, to deal with them and the responses, emotional and otherwise, they engender, and to learn from them. And then move on.

A similar version of this case study was originally published in ACP Observer in January 1996.

REFERENCES

1. Christensen JF, Levison W, Dunn PM. The heart of darkness: the impact of perceived mistakes on physicians. J Gen Intern Med. 1992;7:424-31.
2. Hilfiker D. Facing our mistakes. N Engl J Med. 1984;310:118-22.
3. Leape LL. Error in medicine. JAMA. 1994;272:1851-7.
4. Localio AR, Lawthers AG, Brennan TA, et al. Relation between malpractice claims and adverse events due to negligence: results of the Harvard Medical Practice Study III. N Engl J Med. 1991;325:245-51.
5. Lo B. Disclosing mistakes. In: Lo B, ed. Resolving Ethical Dilemmas: A Guide for Clinicians. Baltimore: William & Wilkins; 1995.
6. American College of Physicians. Ethics Manual, 3rd ed. Ann Intern Med. 1992;117: 947-60.

ANNOTATED BIBLIOGRAPHY

Christensen JF, Levison W, Dunn PM. The heart of darkness: the impact of perceived mistakes on physicians. J Gen Intern Med. 1992;7:424-31.

Physicians were interviewed about a prior mistake and its impact on their life and practice. Among the conclusions of the study were that perceived errors caused emotional distress and that sharing this distress with colleagues varied based on competitiveness as a result of medical training. The authors call for more open discussion of mistakes in practice and training.

Hilfiker D. Facing our mistakes. N Engl J Med. 1984;310:118-22.

A physician shares a significant mistake, its effects, and his thoughts on the need for acknowledgment and discussion of errors among peers.

Leape LL. Error in medicine. JAMA. 1994;272:1851-7.

Looks at the potential for error in medicine, attitudes toward errors and prevention, and possible systems changes to prevent or identify errors in a timely fashion.

Leape LL, Bates DW, Cullen DJ, et al. Systems analysis of adverse drug events. JAMA. 1995;274:35-43.

Identifies and reviews the drug errors that result from systems failures with an eye toward systems changes to improve drug and patient information.

Wu AW, Cavanaugh TA, McPhee SJ, et al. To tell the truth: ethical and practical issues in disclosing medical mistakes to patients. J Gen Intern Med. 1997;12:770-5.

Discusses what doctors should consider in deciding to whether to disclose a mistake. Includes a definition of mistakes, potential benefits, and harms of disclosure to both the patient and the physician, and practical advice to doctors on how to go about disclosing to a patient. Also includes advice on disclosure of mistakes made by other physicians.

16

Sex and the Single Physician
*Commentary and Case History by Janet Weiner, MPH, and
  Susan W. Tolle, MD*

Case History

Leonard Sullivan, age 59, has been one of three general internists in Pumpkin Hills, Wyoming, for the past 30 years. He came to Pumpkin Hills immediately after residency, married a local woman, and raised two children who are now away at college. Dr. Sullivan's wife died of breast cancer a year ago.

Margaret Dinardo, age 60, has spent her life in Pumpkin Hills and has been a patient of Dr. Sullivan's for 20 years. Her husband died 2 years ago, and her children are now married.

Ms. Dinardo returns for her yearly visit with Dr. Sullivan. He finds her in continued good health, renews her prescription for mild osteoarthritis, and schedules her yearly mammogram. Dr. Sullivan reviews the results of his clinical examination, and they talk about general preventive health measures. He notices that he feels uplifted by Ms. Dinardo's presence.

"Enough about me, Leonard," Ms. Dinardo says finally. "How have you been since Diane passed on?"

"It's been difficult, although the children have been a great help," he responds. Ms. Dinardo touches his shoulder, saying, "I know exactly what you mean," and leaves.

About a week later, Ms. Dinardo calls Dr. Sullivan at home and invites him over for dinner. "I bet you don't get many home-cooked meals these days," she says. He accepts, and they spend the evening talking. Dr. Sullivan tells her about his life now, and the trouble he has had coping with the death of his wife. In Margaret Dinardo he finds an understanding and compassionate listener, one who shares

continued on page 100

Case History *continued from page 99*

his experience of losing a spouse. "Thank you, Margaret . . . I feel so much better talking to you," he says.

"Any time, Leonard," she responds. "Call me and maybe we'll catch a movie."

In the next few months, Dr. Sullivan and Ms. Dinardo see each other regularly. They enjoy each other's company and consider their relationship to be an evolution of their long-standing friendship. But Dr. Sullivan begins to notice that he feels romantically inclined toward Ms. Dinardo and wonders if she feels the same. One evening, Ms. Dinardo says, "Leonard, what is the matter with you? You've been fidgeting since you got here." He blurts out that he feels attracted to her romantically, and she replies, "Well, it's about time! I was beginning to think you were just too old for me!"

They kiss passionately, well into the evening. He reluctantly draws away from her and heads toward the door. "I really should be getting home . . . I have a busy day tomorrow at the office. Good night, Margaret."

"Oh, well, duty calls. Good night, Dr. Sullivan," she replies.

He does not sleep, feeling strangely disquieted by the "doctor" in her good night. The next day, too, he is troubled by Ms. Dinardo's use of "Dr. Sullivan." He decides to talk to her about it. "I was always taught that a sexual relationship between a doctor and a patient was wrong," he begins. "If we're going to start something here, maybe you should consider becoming Dr. Voorhees' patient."

Ms. Dinardo reacts with surprise and anger. "Leonard Sullivan, you have been my doctor for 20 years. I trust you—that doesn't just go away because we kissed. How can you even think such a thing?" She refuses to consider seeing another internist. "Now you expect me to give you up as a doctor? You must be kidding!"

What should Dr. Sullivan do?

Commentary

This case study illustrates some of the subtleties and difficulties inherent in the general prohibition against sex between doctor and patient. The prohibition dates back to at least the Hippocratic Oath, which states, "I will come for the benefit of the sick, remaining free of all intentional injustice, of all mischief and in particular of sexual relations with both male and female persons . . ." (1). Although medical and ethical consensus on the prohibition remains intact, recently publicized abuses have brought renewed public and professional attention to the issue.

The American College of Physicians Ethics Manual is clear on this point: "It is unethical for a physician to become sexually involved with a current patient even if the patient initiates or consents to the advances" (2). Likewise, the American Medical Association concludes that "sexual contact or a romantic relationship with a patient concurrent with the physician-patient relationship is unethical" (1). Both organizations also question the wisdom of sexual relationships with former patients. They consider it unethical "if the physician uses or exploits trust, knowledge, emotions, or influence derived from the previous professional relationship" (1).

Four arguments underscore recommendations against sexual contact between physicians and patients:

- **The inequality between the parties.** In patient-physician relationships, patients answer personal questions, reveal sensitive information, and allow the doctor to touch them. This is one-way intimacy; doctors do not ordinarily put themselves in similar positions. True consent by the patient to an intimate relationship is questionable, and initiation of one is suspect, given this inequality.
- **The inherent vulnerability of the patient.** Most patients seeking care are ill and put great faith in the doctor's opinion and advice. The inequality in knowledge and health status puts patients in a vulnerable and dependent position, one that physicians must never exploit.
- **The possibility of betraying the patient's trust.** The social contract between physicians and patients is based on trust; patients trust that the doctor will keep all information confidential and will only use such information to help them. At some point in an intimate relationship, a doctor might use knowledge gained from the therapeutic relationship out of self-interest, or a patient or community might perceive this to be the case. This undermines trust in the profession as a whole.
- **The conflict with the physician's duty to act in the patient's best interests.** In the therapeutic relationship, patients trust that the doctor will keep their interests primary. In a sexual relationship, there are competing and sometimes conflicting interests. The two relationships cannot be reconciled.

For these reasons, sex between doctors and current patients is considered unethical. Ethical concerns are mirrored in legal and regulatory sanctions against this practice. The laws of a number of states consider sexual contact between physicians and patients to be criminal behavior, and such contact is almost universally grounds for action by state licensing boards.

In many ways, our case is not typical of sexual misconduct by doctors who abuse their patients. This is a reality we do not mean to ignore or diminish by the case we have presented. For example, cases of an obstetrician raping a patient under anesthesia, or a psychiatrist having sex with a patient under the guise of therapy, are so obviously wrong that the ethics are obvious. To explore whether the professional ethic holds true in less obvious situations, we have deliberately crafted the most benign, long-standing patient-physician relationship we could imagine.

Despite prohibitions, 5%-10% of all psychiatrists have reported sexual contact with a patient, and it is likely that these figures are similar for other specialists (3). Most of this contact appears clearly exploitative of the patient within the therapeutic relationship. There are well-documented reports of harm to patients from these relationships, which can have devastating effects on their lives and their capacity to trust any other physician. In published studies, 85%-90% of patients experience sexual contact with their physician as damaging, although the data may be biased by selective reporting of more negative reactions (1). Female patients (overwhelmingly the objects of such contact) have been reported to experience guilt, severe distrust of their own judgment, and mistrust of both men and physicians.

We turn now to the more difficult case, like our Dr. Sullivan, in which the physician and patient find themselves attracted to one another in a relationship concurrent with, but apart from, the therapeutic relationship. This can be especially a problem within small rural communities, where a large proportion of the community may be the physician's patients.

On the surface, this case lacks many of the aspects that make doctor-patient sex so disconcerting: Ms. Dinardo does not seem especially vulnerable because she is not acutely or chronically ill. Dr. Sullivan does not seem to be betraying Ms. Dinardo's trust, and their relationship does not seem unequal. Indeed, they seem to step out of their roles in the social context in which they continue to see each other. Should this kind of situation be considered just a matter of consensual activity between two adults? Does the ethical prohibition apply, and if so, why?

Here, the dangers are subtle but still present. Twenty years of a therapeutic relationship may have produced a dependence in Ms. Dinardo that Dr. Sullivan does not recognize. Indeed, Dr. Sullivan's ready willingness to transfer Ms. Dinardo's care, and her extreme objection to being transferred, point to a difference in both perception and power. Physicians and patients may view the sexual relationship quite differently, as well, and may not share the same understanding of the effect of their ongoing or previous therapeutic relationship.

If Dr. Sullivan tries to maintain dual relationships, he would violate a fundamental tenet of medical ethics and physician practice: the promise to keep his patient's interests primary. This violation would occur regardless of the outcome of their intimate relationship. In a sexual relationship, Dr. Sullivan necessarily elevates his own interests to at least the same level as his patient's. He begins to act in his own best interest. Perhaps these interests converge with his patient's and they will live happily ever after. In that instance, Dr. Sullivan's objectivity would be colored, and he should not continue to take care of Ms. Dinardo, for many of the same reasons physicians should not provide ongoing medical care to family members.

But there is no guarantee of future happiness. One of the strongest arguments against doctor-patient sex is that it might not work out forever. Dr. Sullivan and Ms. Dinardo could embark upon an intimate relationship that falls apart after a length of time. Perhaps the breakup would not be without rancor. It is likely that Dr. Sullivan and Ms. Dinardo could not continue a trusting clinical relationship, and one or both would want to sever the professional ties. In that scenario, it is clearer that the patient's interests had not remained primary, which had led to a conflict of interest.

Therefore, in either scenario, it would not be in Ms. Dinardo's best interests to remain Dr. Sullivan's patient if they want to become more intimate. It would also not be in Dr. Sullivan's best interests. He risks losing his license if reported to the state board, and he risks the confidence of his other patients and the community if he becomes intimate with a current patient. Knowing this, it is important to transfer her care before they begin an intimate relationship.

Even former patients may continue to feel dependent or vulnerable, and Dr. Sullivan should carefully assess this possibility (consultation with an objective colleague may help). The danger to former patients of a relationship with their psychiatrist has been recognized by criminal or civil laws in a number of states (4). Most of these laws dictate a 1- to 2-year interval as an appropriate safeguard against abuse. Of course, internists may not face the same issues of transference and power imbalance as psychiatrists. The delay necessary to protect a patient will vary with the people involved and the nature, extent, and intensity of the prior professional relationship.

A similar version of this case study was originally published in ACP Observer in July/August 1992.

REFERENCES

1. Council on Ethical and Judicial Affairs, American Medical Association. Sexual misconduct in the practice of medicine. JAMA. 1991;266:2741-5.
2. American College of Physicians. Ethics Manual, 3rd ed. Ann Intern Med. 1992; 117:947-60.
3. Gartrell N, Herman J, Olarte S, et al. Psychiatrist-patient sexual contact. Results of a national survey. I: Prevalence. Am J Psychiatry. 1986;143:1126-31.
4. Applebaum PS, Jorgenson L. Psychotherapist-patient sexual contact after termination of treatment: an analysis and a proposal. Am J Psychiatry. 1991;148:1466-73.

ANNOTATED BIBLIOGRAPHY

Council on Ethical and Judicial Affairs, American Medical Association. Sexual misconduct in the practice of medicine. JAMA. 1991;266:2741-5.

Explains why physicians should not have sex with patients and, in certain situations, with former patients. Encourages ethics education about physician-patient sex and rigorous reporting of sexual misconduct.

Dehlendorf CE, Wolfe SM. Physicians disciplined for sex-related offenses. JAMA. 1998; 279:1883-8.

Finds that discipline of physicians for sex-related offenses increased from 1989 to 1996 and orders against licenses were more severe than for non-sex-related offenses. The total number of physicians disciplined for sexual offenses remained low, however, and those disciplined often continued or returned to practice.

Johnson SH. Judicial review of disciplinary action for sexual misconduct in the practice of medicine. JAMA. 1993;270:1596-600.

A lawyer looks at the legal implications of a professional ethic prohibiting sexual contact between physician and patient, plus early court cases.

White GE, Coverdale JA, Thomson AN. Can one be a good doctor and have a sexual relationship with one's patient? Fam Pract. 1994;11:389-93.

Participants in a study of primary care physicians offer a range of definitions regarding sexual contact, social contact, and who constitutes a patient. Authors call for appropriate guidelines for physicians and better educational efforts through the teaching of medical students and continuing medical education.

Part III

MEDICINE'S COLLECTIVE OBLIGATIONS

No man is an island. No physician is an island in the sea of medicine.

In addition to their primary duties to their individual patients, physicians have duties to patients collectively, to other physicians, and to society. Some of these duties are considered in Part III. Chapters look at nursing home care, research ethics in the doctor's office, immigrant reporting, physician participation in executions, and the ethical (as distinct from the legal) duty to treat poor patients and HIV-infected and AIDS patients. Also explored are the physician's obligations regarding an impaired colleague, the responsibilities and mistakes of medical residents, and disagreements between residents and attendings.

17

Nursing Home "Dumps": Should You Go Along or Speak Up?

Commentary and Case History by Joanne Lynn, MD

Case History

Mrs. Smith was back in the emergency room. The 88-year-old nursing home resident had been brought into the hospital every few weeks for the past several months with fevers and other complications. She was hearing-impaired and suffered from dementia. Delirious in the unfamiliar surroundings of the hospital, she was yelling and generally disruptive.

The nurses started the work-up and the admissions process. Although the house staff team was not pleased to see another "nursing home dump" admission, they started an intravenous line for fluids and antibiotics, checked a chest X-ray, and gave Mrs. Smith a thorough examination. After a 3-day stay in the hospital, the patient returned to the nursing home with a diagnosis of urinary tract infection and a prescription for oral antibiotics.

A few days later, a medical student who had helped care for Mrs. Smith encountered her at the nursing home at the beginning of a medicine rotation. The student was surprised to see her former patient smiling and cheerful, looking at pictures that a group of elementary school children visiting the home had drawn for her. It was hard to believe that this was the same person who had been in such obvious distress in the emergency room just a few days earlier.

After spending some time in the nursing home, the medical student came to realize that it was a valuable community for the severely ill and disabled, not an inferior version of a hospital. For

continued on page 108

Case History *continued from page 107*

patients like Mrs. Smith, the environment was clearly much more appropriate.

During her visit, the student encountered Dr. Welby, one of the physicians who had treated Mrs. Smith at the teaching hospital. During her conversation with him, she asked, "When Mrs. Smith gets a fever, are you sure it does her good to send her to the hospital?"

"No, I don't think it does," Dr. Welby answered.

The student persisted: "Then why do it?"

"There are lots of reasons, but I don't like any of them," Dr. Welby replied. "She would probably do better if I could keep her here. She wouldn't get skin breakdowns or tears, she would never be restrained, and she would be among people who know and care about her. But we just can't afford it. The nursing home gets paid the same per day to treat a patient with antibiotics and one without, and Mrs. Smith usually needs more than $100 a day in antibiotics alone. The nursing home gets no additional income for a day when she needs repeated monitoring and assessments.

"When she is in the hospital," he continued, "I get paid, the nursing home doesn't run up costs, and everyone does well, except perhaps Mrs. Smith. She has no family to advocate for her or even to accept less aggressive medical treatment in order to keep her more comfortable. So we just keep doing this. And it's not just Mrs. Smith. We hospitalize dozens of people from here every month, and with most of them we're caught in the same bind. I don't like it, but it's the best I can do. I know we could do better if we kept her here, but we can't afford that."

The student was upset at what was happening to Mrs. Smith. She realized that her colleagues were not interested in addressing nursing home "dumps" and, although she knew that something was wrong, she was not sure that she could fault Dr. Welby.

Commentary

Increasingly, physicians are complaining that the systems in which they work do not best serve the interests of patients. Particularly when it comes to caring for patients in nursing homes, many say, the incentives seem to run counter to good medical care.

As physicians, we sometimes see the shortcomings all too clearly. We can make an occasional accommodation to keep a system functioning, but can we accept recurring inadequacy? If we are unhappy with the situation, what can we do about it?

Although the doctor in this case study is functioning in a deficient system whose failures are self-perpetuating, a good physician must do something to try to improve such a situation. It may be difficult to decide exactly what to do, but that should not obscure the physician's obligation to speak up and try to improve a flawed system.

To define what the physician should do to help bring about change, it's helpful to consider what a good system of care would look like. For one, it would be able to care for many acutely ill nursing home residents on-site, and it would encourage residents to make hospitalization and resuscitation plans in advance. In addition, hospital care for this population would cause fewer iatrogenic complications, and the payment system would not punish nursing homes for providing acute care for their patients.

With that in mind, there are several steps the physician can take when faced with this kind of situation. For example, one possible approach would be to go to nursing home administrators and explore the idea of caring for a few of the frailest patients at the nursing home, without transfer. Physicians could use such an opportunity to see if it is possible to provide adequate care in these instances in the nursing home without running up too much of a bill.

Another avenue is to explore having a local hospice provide on-site care. Though changes in Medicare regulations may soon alter the situation, Medicare hospice can usually be made available to nursing home residents. The hospice gets paid almost the same daily rate as for patients at home, though for patients who are also relying upon Medicaid, that payment is routed through the hospice program, which then pays the nursing facility. The hospice benefit is only available when the two programs have a written agreement that meets certain requirements, so coordination and advance planning are essential.

Talking to the emergency room medical staff and hospital administration may also yield fruitful suggestions on how to improve the care of nursing home patients. For example, the emergency room staff might welcome clarifications to routine advance directives so they can more easily understand and trust the written forms that the patient brings. The hospital might also be willing to move a nursing home resident to a regular hospital bed more quickly to limit the hazards of falls and skin breakdown that so often occur in the emergency room. Perhaps hospital physicians could also take the lead in talking to a patient's family about re-hospitalization for long-term chronic problems.

Physicians could also collect data on the frequency and outcomes of situations where nursing home residents are transferred to hospital emergency rooms. It might turn out, for example, that the problem transfers are mostly confined to one nursing home, or involve patients with a particular set of conditions, and responses could be tailored to those situations. Measuring the frequency of transfers may help galvanize nursing home leadership into taking these situations seriously.

Playing an active role in advance care planning in the nursing home for hospitalization and resuscitation could also help to ameliorate the problem. Many patients this frail, or their families, are willing to take their chances with the treatments they can get in their nursing facility, and they should have the opportunity to make that desire known. Even those who want more aggressive treatment often have limits that they can articulate: a time-limited trial on a respirator, for example. Knowing about such considerations in advance would be helpful and would allow physicians to tailor care to the patient and family in an efficient and a sensitive way.

An even more direct tactic would be to approach the local Medicaid carrier to find out what accommodations it might be able to provide. For example, the carrier might be willing to subsidize advance care planning or care management. Physicians could also ask the local quality review organization to study the procedures and suggest possible ways of improvement.

Ultimately, working to help mobilize political forces to change Medicare and Medicaid reimbursements is a key to achieving better care. Physicians can start by writing letters to their representatives and professional societies.

Obviously, physicians can't spend all of their time on this issue; it is likely to be just one of many problems that demand their attention. Moreover, not every nursing home can take on the level of care that such improvements might require. Change of any sort may be troubling or threatening to colleagues, and even strong efforts by physicians may prove ineffective.

Physicians, however, are often in a unique position to identify problems, and they have real power to effect change. A physician's ethical obligation as a patient advocate extends beyond individual patients (1). Physicians also have a responsibility to help improve health care delivery systems that disadvantage or devalue patient care (1-4). Only then can physicians serve their patients and communities well. If they are not part of the continuing improvement of our systems of care, the problems are likely to continue.

A similar version of this case study was originally published in ACP Observer in October 1999.

References

1. American College of Physicians. Ethics Manual, 4th ed. Ann Intern Med. 1998;128: 576-94.
2. Pellegrino ED. Ethics. JAMA. 1994;271:1668-70.
3. Povar G, Moreno J. Hippocrates and the health maintenance organization: a discussion of ethical issues. Ann Intern Med. 1988;109:419-24.
4. Sulmasy DP. Physicians, cost control, and ethics. Ann Intern Med. 1992;116:920-6.

18

Industry-Sponsored Trials and Community Doctors

Commentary and Case History by David Casarett, MD,
Lois Snyder, JD, and Jason Karlawish, MD

Case History

Drs. Smith and Jones, senior partners of Internal Medicine Associates, have never before done office-based industry-sponsored drug research. Recently, Dr. Brown from DrugCo invited them to serve as co-investigators in a randomized double-blind clinical trial of a new medication to treat type 2 diabetes. It is the last trial DrugCo needs to complete before applying for FDA review and approval of the drug.

Rather than going to University Hospital's Institutional Review Board, DrugCo has arranged for a contract research organization (CRO) to manage the whole trial, including institutional review board (IRB) review, study design, data analysis, article preparation, and FDA applications.

Subjects who enroll will be randomly selected to receive either one or two doses of the new drug or a placebo for 6 months. The prospect that some of his patients will get the placebo, not treatment, for that length of time concerns Dr. Smith. Subjects cannot take any other oral drugs for diabetes.

DrugCo will pay the doctors $3000 per enrolled subject and will pay for all study-related care. In addition, if Drs. Smith and Jones enroll 10 subjects in 3 months, they will receive an additional $5000. (Dr. Jones is a bit surprised by the level of these fees and worries about the practice becoming dependent on this kind of income.) Finally, a number of papers will be published from the study, and Drs. Smith and Jones are welcome to participate as co-authors.

continued on page 113

> **Case History** *continued from page 112*
>
> After taking courses in evidence-based medicine and putting their practice database online, Drs. Smith and Jones are definitely interested in office-based clinical research. They serve an urban population that includes many chronically ill, elderly, and low-income patients and believe that better data are needed to substantiate best practices for this population. Moreover, the trial is attractive because it promises free medication, and many of their patients have been hard hit by drug costs. However, the partners want to think through the ramifications before going forward.

Commentary

Drs. Smith and Jones are carefully considering participating in a study in order to advance sound, clinic-based effectiveness research. A decision to participate will have ramifications for them, their patients, their patient-physician relationships, and their practice.

Physicians who do research involving their patients have a dual role and must be aware of potential conflicts between what is best for the patient-subject and what is optimal for the conduct of the research. However, the lines between clinician and researcher can become fuzzy, as can the lines between patient and subject (1,2).

Nevertheless, physician-investigators must consider their role as physicians first and as investigators second, and they should ensure that research they participate in is ethically conducted (3). Therefore, as they consider this opportunity, Drs. Smith and Jones should evaluate the validity and value of the research, the ethical and scientific review that it has undergone, and compensation and authorship issues.

Validity

Drs. Smith and Jones' first consideration should be the study's validity. A study is scientifically valid if it answers the questions that it asks (4). The study in question would be considered valid if it has a large enough universe of subjects to provide statistically significant results, and if the intervention and measurement techniques are sufficient to settle a research hypothesis. For instance, the goal of the study could be to prove that the new medication is more effective than a similar product.

Validity is a threshold requirement for all research because it is unethical to expose human subjects to risks in studies that peer reviewers agree cannot adequately answer a research question (5). Because of this peer-review element, assessing the study's validity might be beyond the scope of what Drs. Smith and Jones can answer independently.

If the study were funded by the National Institutes of Health or another institution that requires careful peer review, Drs. Smith and Jones could rely on this process as an assessment of validity. But the study they are considering is privately funded, with no such process of external review. However, they might look at the reputations of the study's investigators and advisory panel. If they are still unsure of the study's scientific quality, they could seek permission to send the protocol for informal, independent review.

To find a reviewer, they can contact medical schools, which may be able to recommend a faculty member with relevant experience. If serious questions arise about the study's validity, further considerations are irrelevant. Drs. Smith and Jones should not participate.

Value

If they believe the study meets initial validity criteria, they should next carefully consider the study's value. A study's scientific value is based on the relevance or importance of its results (4). Good research is designed to produce knowledge that ultimately proves "important,"(6) "fruitful"(7) or "valuable"(8). Unlike assessments of validity, judging value does not yield a yes/no answer, but a ranking on a continuum.

A useful test for Dr. Smith and Jones might be to ask whether a study's results have the potential to change their practice immediately or in the future. If the study seeks determine whether a new medication is superior to an existing one, for example, it may offer considerable value. On the other hand, if DrugCo is seeking to simply obtain approval for a "me-too" medication that offers no advantages over currently available therapies, its value is suspect.

A study's value also depends upon who will benefit from the results. Drs. Smith and Jones believe their patients lack the resources to pay for medications. Therefore, it seems likely that they will also be unable to afford the study medication if and when it is approved. The study's value may not apply to them.

A lack of value, unlike a lack of validity, should not necessarily cause Drs. Smith and Jones to reject the study. However, they should view it with muted enthusiasm.

Ethical Review

Drs. Smith and Jones should next consider carefully the processes of ethical review that the study has undergone. At a minimum, most research carried out in the United States must go through review by an interdisciplinary IRB or meet stringent criteria for exemption from review (6). IRBs evaluate several aspects of a proposed study, including its risks, benefits, consent process, confidentiality issues, recruitment practices, and the importance of the knowledge to be gained (6).

If an institution has an IRB, as University Hospital likely does, that IRB should review the protocol. Indeed, if University Hospital accepts federal money for research, it is required to adhere to regulations governing the conduct of research, including IRB review (6). Local review is important because a committee whose members are drawn from the institution and the community are best prepared to assess a study's risks and benefit in light of the unique needs and concerns of that institution's patient population.

For all of these reasons, Drs. Smith and Jones should make sure that the protocol is reviewed by their hospital's IRB. "All proposed clinical research, regardless of the source of support, should be approved by the local IRB to ensure that the research plans are reasonable and that the research participants are adequately protected" (3).

If clinicians are not affiliated with an institution that has an IRB, they must rely on the IRB affiliated with the CRO to provide ethical oversight. To expedite trials, industry has increasingly used CROs and site-management organizations, rather than academic medical centers. In fact, industry funding for trials in academic centers fell from 80% in 1991 to 40% in 1998 (9).

Although this CRO-based review process should be objective, it lacks understanding of the local patient population required for adequate review. An outside IRB may not scrutinize studies as carefully as a local IRB, which needs to maintain community relations and patient trust. Therefore, clinicians who participate in research should be aware that they will have to take on the role of the local IRB to some degree, particularly by ensuring that the consent information is appropriate for their patients. Clinicians without access to an IRB may wish to contract with a nearby academic medical center IRB that is willing to review protocols for a fee that could then be billed to the CRO.

Compensation

Drs. Smith and Jones should also seek advice from local or distant IRBs regarding their other concerns, particularly the compensation they have been offered. A reasonable rule of thumb is that payments should be commensurate with the time and effort spent and the expenses incurred in recruitment. Compensation above this level is pure profit, and constitutes, or could be perceived to constitute, a conflict of interest. Providing finder's fees to individual physicians for referring patients to a study "generates an unethical conflict of interest" (3). Drs. Smith and Jones should refuse the offer of a bonus for active recruitment.

This recommendation reflects commonly accepted standards for referrals in clinical care. For instance, if a laboratory approached Drs. Smith and Jones and offered them payments for each patient they referred, they would no doubt refuse, citing guidelines about improper business relationships and fee-splitting (3,10-12). The same is true for this study.

Drs. Smith and Jones should seek advice from the IRB about the added expenses of trial recruitment and follow up (which may be substantial) and for advice about proper compensation. Not all IRBs consider recruitment practices and incentives to be within the scope of their review (13). Some specify what is permissible and what is not, and some require investigators to disclose any potential conflicts of interest (1).

Placebo Controls

Another big concern Drs. Smith and Jones might have about the study is the use of placebo controls. The World Medical Association Declaration of Helsinki on Ethical Principles for Medical Research Involving Human Subjects exhorts researchers to test against the "best current prophylactic, diagnostic, and therapeutic methods" and to only use placebo or no treatment in studies where no proven method exists (14). Human subject research advocates see this principle as a way to protect subjects' welfare, especially for research done in developing countries.

Those who support the wider use of placebo-controlled trials cite the scientific necessity of such studies in certain circumstances. They contend that, as long as alternatives are fully disclosed, the ethical appropriateness of placebos should be determined based on whether the subject will be harmed by deferring therapy (15,16).

Authorship

This study raises other concerns beyond the purview of most IRBs, such as the CRO's offer of authorship opportunities. Although it is not, strictly speaking, an issue of research ethics, this offer involves broader issues of professionalism and scientific propriety.

In general, subject recruitment alone does not warrant authorship. Instead, authorship requires involvement in developing a study's conception and design, analyzing and interpreting results, drafting or revising the article's intellectual content, and approving the final version (17). Drs. Smith and Jones have not been involved in conception and design. Unless they are invited and agree to participate in interpreting and reporting the study results, their level of participation is unlikely to warrant authorship in many medical journals.

Making a Decision

The ethical conduct of research, like the scientific conduct of research, requires careful consideration, planning, and attention to detail. Clinicians who are interested in contributing to research should spend some time learning about the responsible conduct of research, perhaps through courses now required by the NIH at most academic medical centers. Clinicians should also identify resources like IRBs, ethics centers, and experienced investigators that can advise them.

A similar version of this case study was originally published in ACP Observer in March 2001.

References

1. Department of Health and Human Services, Office of the Inspector General. Recruiting Human Subjects: Sample Guidelines for Practice. 2000. Publication no. OEI-01-97-00196.
2. Appelbaum P, Roth L, Lidz C, et al. False hopes and best data: consent to research and the therapeutic misconception. Hastings Center Report. 1987;17:20-4.
3. American College of Physicians. Ethics Manual, 4th ed. Ann Intern Med. 1998;128: 576-94.
4. Freedman B. Scientific value and validity as ethical requirements for research: a proposed explication. IRB. 1987;9:7-10.
5. Rutstein DR. The ethical design of human experiments. In: Freund PA, ed. Experimentation with Human Subjects. New York: George Braziller; 1970:383-401.
6. Department of Health and Human Services. Protection of Human Subjects. Title 45, Part 46: Revised. Code of Federal Regulation. 18 June 1991.
7. The Nuremberg Code. In: Brody H. The Ethics of Biomedical Research: An International Perspective. New York: Oxford University Press; 1947:213.
8. Freedman B. Placebo-controlled trials and the logic of clinical purpose. IRB. 1990; 12:1-6.
9. Bodenheimer T. Uneasy alliance: clinical investigators and the pharmaceutical industry. N Engl J Med. 2000;342:1539-44.
10. Thompson DF. Understanding financial conflicts of interest. N Engl J Med. 1993; 329:573-6.
11. Relman AS. Dealing with conflicts of interest. N Engl J Med. 1985;313:749-51.
12. American Medical Association. Conflicts of Interest. Council on Ethical and Judicial Affairs, Report A (I-86); 1986.

13. Department of Health and Human Services, Office of the Inspector General. Recruiting Human Subjects: Pressures in Industry-Sponsored Clinical Research. 2000. Publication no. OEI-01-97-00195.

14. World Medical Association. Declaration of Helsinki. Ethical principles for medical research involving human subjects. JAMA. 2000;283:3043-5.

15. Ellenberg SS, Temple R. Placebo-controlled trials and active-control trials in the evaluation of new treatments. Part 1. Ethical and scientific issues. Ann Intern Med. 2000;133:455-63.

16. Ellenberg SS, Temple R. Placebo-controlled trials and active-control trials in the evaluation of new treatments. Part 2. Practical issues and specific cases. Ann Intern Med. 2000;133:464-70.

17. International Committee of Medical Journal Editors. Uniform requirements for manuscripts submitted to biomedical journals. JAMA. 1997;277:927-34.

ANNOTATED BIBLIOGRAPHY

American Medical Association Council on Ethical and Judicial Affairs. Opinion 8.031, Conflicts of Interest: Biomedical Research. Code of Medical Ethics: Current Opinions. Chicago: American Medical Association; 2000:69.

Guidelines from the American Medical Association on clinical research and conflicts of interest.

Marquis D. How to resolve an ethical dilemma concerning randomized clinical trials. N Engl J Med. 1999;341:691-3.

Strategies are suggested regarding the enrollment of patients in randomized clinical trials, particularly when the physician has an opinion about which treatment is better.

Miller FG, Rosenstein DL, DeRenzo EG. Professional integrity in clinical research. JAMA. 1998;280:1449-54.

Examines the conflict between the physician's role as both clinician and investigator, and the concept of "therapeutic misconception." Emphasizes the need for education to promote professional integrity in clinical research.

Vastag B. Helsinki discord? A controversial declaration. JAMA. 2000;284:2983-5.

Discusses the fifth revision of the Declaration of Helsinki and reactions to the position on the use of placebos in clinical trials.

World Medical Association. Declaration of Helsinki. Ethical principles for medical research involving human subjects. JAMA. 2000;283:3043-5.

The World Medical Association identifies ethical principles to be considered during human subjects research.

19

Checking Up on Immigrants: A Job for Physicians?

Commentary by Peter A. Ubel, MD
Case History by Bernard Lo, MD, and Lois Snyder, JD

Case History

California internist Frank James has just concluded an examination of a new patient, 33-year-old Joseph Lopez. Mr. Lopez complains of fever and has also been experiencing night sweats and weight loss for the past month or so. "Are you coughing?" asks Dr. James. "Yes," the patient responds. When Dr. James asks if anyone else in the family is coughing or seems sick, Mr. Lopez falls silent and looks scared. "I smoke," he says. "Coughing from smoke."

Dr. James doesn't agree. He suspects tuberculosis and believes Mr. Lopez needs evaluation for the possibility of a co-infection with HIV. He asks Mr. Lopez if he has had a tuberculin skin test before; the patient says he doesn't think so. Dr. James performs the skin test. He tells Mr. Lopez he wants him to go to Memorial General Hospital for more tests, and orders a sputum culture and chest X-ray. He learns that the patient has no insurance.

"No hospital," says Mr. Lopez in broken English. "187." Dr. James understands Mr. Lopez to be referencing California's Proposition 187, which restricts non-emergency medical care for undocumented immigrants and requires that they be reported to the state and the Immigration and Naturalization Service if they seek care at a "publicly funded health care facility."

"Are you in this country legally?" Dr. James asks the patient, anticipating he will say no, given that he had not previously had a skin test. Instead, there is no response. "Well," Dr. James continues,

continued on page 120

Case History *continued from page 119*

"Proposition 187 has been tied up in the courts. No patients are having their immigration status checked, and no one is being reported to INS. I don't think we need to worry about 187 right now." "No hospital," Mr. Lopez repeats. Dr. James says he will find out more about Proposition 187 and emphasizes the importance of the hospital tests. He asks the patient to have the receptionist schedule another appointment for next week.

Later that day, Dr. James discovers that Mr. Lopez did not make a follow-up appointment. The patient paid cash for that day's visit and when asked about follow-up, he responded "187."

Commentary

The case presented here describes a man who clearly needs medical attention but fears that he will be thrown out of the country if he seeks care. It shows how laws like Proposition 187 might harm patients by encouraging them to avoid health care even when they have curable illnesses.

Proposition 187 has the potential to hurt the health of individuals, but it may also harm the doctor-patient relationship. Patients need to know that they can trust their physician to look out for their interests and to maintain confidentiality with few exceptions. This trust cannot be maintained if patients come to regard their physicians as police. This holds true for undocumented immigrants, who would fear being expelled from the country as a result of seeking care, and for legal immigrants, who could find physicians hesitant to provide care to patients they fear might be undocumented immigrants.

California's Proposition 187 was passed in the midst of a large state budget deficit that led to reductions in state Medicaid funding and pressure to reduce health care and other spending for undocumented aliens. Of all states, California has sustained the largest burden of costs for the provision of health care to undocumented aliens. In 1993, the state spent an estimated $389 million out of $731 million of total state and federal Medicaid funds on emergency care for undocumented aliens. (The next closest states: New York, Illinois, and Texas, spent $23, $19.7, and $19.4 million, respectively [1].) This level of spending contributed to the vote tally; 59% of California residents voted to pass Proposition 187.

The California Medical Association and the American Medical Association opposed Proposition 187 on the grounds that it would endanger public health and violate the confidentiality of the doctor-patient relationship. This raises an important question: Should medical professionals or society as a whole determine professional norms?

Tensions exist between the medical profession's need to establish ethical standards and society's need to regulate the profession. Since the time of Hippocrates, physicians may have taken the lead in creating ethics codes that guide physician behavior. But legal standards also have improved the medical profession's moral standards: the law, for instance, was instrumental in improving standards of informed consent in medical practice.

In many cases, however, society and the medical profession have different ideas about what physicians ought to do. Debates about whether physicians should assist in patient suicide, be involved in capital punishment, or discuss options like abortion illustrate the tension between societal and medical views of physicians' professional duties.

Proposition 187 is the latest example of this tension. The public has asked health care providers to collect and disclose information about patients that has nothing to do with the individual's medical status. The vulnerability of the sick is used as a tool for furthering a completely unrelated goal: finding illegal aliens and expelling them from the country.

Checking the immigration status of patients is not an appropriate function for physicians and other health care providers and is an interference with the doctor-patient relationship. Technically, under Proposition 187 publicly funded health care facilities, not physicians like Dr. James, have to report undocumented aliens. Publicly funded health care facilities are defined as those "to which persons are admitted for a 24-hour stay or longer." But while Dr. James can treat and need not report Mr. Lopez, the patient also needs hospital care.

There is also concern that facilities may check the immigration status of legal immigrants based on their ethnicity. This could lead to discrimination, with immigrants from Europe receiving care and immigrants from Latin American or other countries receiving scrutiny. It is hard to imagine any of this improving the doctor-patient relationship.

In addition, the case shows how Proposition 187 might harm the public health, because the patients avoiding care may be infected with a disease like tuberculosis and spread it throughout the community. This would clearly interfere with the profession's mandate that "physicians must fulfill the profession's collective responsibility to be advocates for the health of the public" as well as that of individual patients (2). The law also violates the tenet that a physician may not discriminate against a class or category of patients by denying appropriate care (2,3).

While it is true that physicians are legally required to report all cases of tuberculosis to the public health department, this breach of confidentiality is acceptable because it serves the public health. However, physicians cannot report cases of tuberculosis that they do not see, and if people with tuberculosis refuse to see a physician, the spread of tuberculosis will increase, harming public health.

California voters have passed a law that asks physicians to do things that contradict their most basic duties to protect the health of the individual patient and the public. Society has helped improve the medical profession in many ways, but in the case of Proposition 187, physicians could be faced with a law that is harmful both to the public health and to the ethics of the profession. (Proposition 187 remains blocked by court order until litigation is resolved.)

With the privilege of practicing medicine comes responsibility. Physicians must remember that they "are morally as well as legally accountable, and the two may not be concordant . . . Physicians must keep in mind the distinctions and potential conflicts between legal and ethical obligations when making clinical decisions" (2). Until the status of Proposition 187 is resolved, and even afterwards, physicians should do everything they can to take care of patients, regardless of whether they are legal or illegal immigrants.

A similar version of this case study was originally published in ACP Observer in October 1996.

REFERENCES

1. Urban Institute. Fiscal Impacts of Undocumented Aliens. Washington, DC: Urban Institute; September 1994.
2. American College of Physicians. Ethics Manual, 3rd ed. Ann Intern Med.1992; 117:947-60.
3. Snyder L, Weiner J. Ethics and medicaid patients. In: Snyder L, ed. Ethical Choices: Case Studies for Medical Practice. Philadelphia: American College of Physicians; 1996.

ANNOTATED BIBLIOGRAPHY

Bilchik GS. No easy answers. Hosp Health Net. 2001;May:59-60.

Discussion of how hospitals bear the costs for the care of illegal immigrants in the United States.

20

Should Doctors Participate in Executions?

Commentary and Case History by Kim M. Thorburn, MD, MPH,
and Janet Weiner, MPH

Case History

Brad Gorden is an internist who is chief physician at a large state prison where executions are carried out by intravenous infusion of lethal doses of three drugs: sodium pentobarbital, pancuronium bromide, and potassium chloride. There have been two executions by lethal injection during the 5 years that Dr. Gorden has worked at the prison.

Neither state law nor administrative regulation requires physician participation in the lethal-injection executions. A Board of Pharmacy waiver permits the warden to buy the drugs at calculated doses according to a formula developed by the state-run school of pharmacy. Pharmacy technicians prepare the intravenous solution containing the drugs, and medical technicians prepare the intravenous lines and perform the venipuncture. Executions are carried out in the early morning.

During the two previous executions, Dr. Gorden elected to be at the prison but not in the execution chamber. He stayed in the institution as a favor to the warden, who had indicated that the doctor's presence would have a settling effect on staff and that the prison would be better prepared in case the other prisoners inflicted injuries upon themselves or reacted violently to the execution. After each of the executions, Dr. Gorden joined the chaplain and the execution team for a debriefing in the warden's office.

Dr. Gorden continued his practice of being at the prison for the third execution. As with the previous executions, he knew the con-

continued on page 124

Case History *continued from page 123*

demned man well as a patient. The prisoner, William Jones, was a long-time heroin user who was convicted of murdering a convenience store cashier during a robbery.

The telephone rang as Dr. Gorden sat in his office in the prison health care facility thinking of Mr. Jones's imminent execution. He picked up the receiver and noticed that it was early to be receiving the call for the post-execution conference. As he surmised, there was a problem. The caller reported that, after numerous attempts, the technicians had been unable to establish intravenous access. Mr. Jones was agitated and had pleaded, "Can't you get someone in here to do this right?" Dr. Gorden recalled that once, when he had ordered some laboratory analysis on Mr. Jones, he was forced to collect the blood from a femoral puncture because neither he nor the medical technicians had been able to access a peripheral venous site. The warden was now ordering Dr. Gorden to come to the execution chamber to assist.

How should Dr. Gorden respond?

Commentary

The issue of physician participation in executions strikes at the heart of our identities as physicians on three distinct levels: as providers of medical care to individuals, as employees of institutions, and as members of a profession that holds the societal trust.

The principles of beneficence and non-maleficence ("first, do no harm") have led many medical organizations, including American College of Physicians (ACP), to positions prohibiting physician participation in carrying out the death penalty. The third edition of the ACP Ethics Manual states: "Participation by physicians in the execution of prisoners, except to certify death, is unethical" (1).

Through the resolution process, ACP has prompted the American Medical Association to call upon states to codify this prohibition in law or regulation (2), and in response to the ACP-authored resolution, the AMA issued a report reaffirming that it is unethical for physicians to participate in executions and specifying what actions constitute participation. The report defines physician participation as:

- Action which would directly cause the death of the condemned, assist another individual to directly cause the death of the condemned, or cause an execution to be carried out.
- Prescribing or administering tranquilizers and other psychotropic agents and medications, monitoring vital signs on site or remotely, attending or observing an execution as a physician, and giving technical advice during an execution.
- In executions where lethal injection is used, selecting injection sites; starting intravenous lines as a port for injection; prescribing, preparing, administering, or supervising injection drugs or their dose or types; inspecting, testing or maintaining lethal injection devices; and consulting with or supervising lethal injection personnel.

The report also defines what is not considered to be physician participation:

- Testifying as to the competence to stand trial or medical relevance of evidence.
- Certifying death if death has already been declared by another person.
- Witnessing an execution in a non-professional capacity or without participating at the request of the condemned.
- Relieving the acute suffering of the condemned while awaiting execution.

Our case points out the conflicts that may arise because of absolute prohibition. Mr. Jones is probably suffering from the botched preparations for the execution. Dr. Gorden may feel torn. He wants to respond to Mr. Jones' distress, but he needs to avoid participating in the execution. Dr. Gorden possesses the skills to complete the preparations and perhaps diminish Mr. Jones' suffering. It might be argued that Dr. Gorden's intervention at this stage would be an application of the beneficence principle. Further, since Mr. Jones asked for help, the doctor may have a duty to give some weight to the "patient's" request, perhaps even to honor it.

This argument is not persuasive, although Mr. Jones' distress is quite real. Responding to Mr. Jones' request would involve using medical skills to expedite an objective—the execution—that is contrary to the profession's mission. Placing a central venous catheter clearly involves complicity in killing Mr. Jones. Lessening his suffering during the execution process, for example, by administering a sedative in the execution chamber, does not excuse responsibility for the final outcome. Nazi doctors sometimes used the concept of expediency to justify their application of medical skills to mass killings.

However, Dr. Gorden is an employee as well as a physician. He works for the warden, who expects his presence in the institution while executions are being carried out. The warden has ordered Dr. Gorden to come to the execution chamber to assist. Does Dr. Gorden have an obligation to serve the warden and the institution?

The warden is responsible for the smooth operation of the prison. In our case, his responsibility is to preside over a legally sanctioned killing, which, optimally, proceeds neatly from beginning to end. When a problem develops during the execution, the warden chooses to turn to the employee who has the necessary skills to solve it.

To understand the conflict here, we must review the reason that Dr. Gorden is employed at the prison. The warden is obligated to provide medical care to the inmates of his institution. Because the warden himself does not have the necessary skills, he has hired Dr. Gorden, and entrusts him to fulfill this fiduciary responsibility to provide medical care to the inmates.

In order for Dr. Gorden to fulfill this duty, he must be able to establish and maintain professional relationships with the inmates as patients. The physician-patient relationship is grounded in trust, which can be eroded when the physician has responsibilities to two parties: the patient and the institution. The doctor must do what he can to protect his relationships with patients. Using medical skills to kill a person would be detrimental to his relationship with patients because it would be clear that Dr. Gorden is willing to serve purposes that are diametrically opposed to patients' interests and good medical care. The warden and institution are not served if Dr. Gorden cannot meet his primary obligation of patient care because inmates do not trust him as a physician.

The problem arose, in part, because Dr. Gorden complied with the warden's request that he stay in the institution during executions. The warden's reasons have nothing to do with the physician's job responsibilities. Prison guards are responsible for security; their presence is necessary to try to prevent violence. The doctor would only be responsible for responding to any medical consequences of such acts should they occur. Dr. Gorden's availability to the execution team staff could also compromise his relationship with prisoner patients. Unlike inmates, correctional officers have other sources of medical care. In order for Dr. Gorden to be effective as a medical caregiver, prisoners must know that Dr. Gorden is there for them and not the staff, who are often viewed as adversaries.

Applications for Other Employed Physicians

Although these arguments seem specific to prison settings, they can be generalized in part to other institutions. As employees of the military or in factories, physicians must fulfill their responsibility to provide medical care in the context of distinct institutional objectives. These objectives may conflict with the delivery of medical care.

In these settings, it is the physician employee's role to provide and advocate for care that is untainted by other goals. The fundamental tenets of the medical profession—beneficence, patient advocacy, and trust—must not be compromised by conflicted institutional objectives. It may be useful for the physician to emphasize these tenets before employment, when interviewing or negotiating with the institution.

At the same time, the physician can gain a better understanding of the institution's objectives in hiring a physician, and may be more able to gauge any constraints that might be placed on providing medical care. For example, a company physician may be expected to break patient confidentiality to disclose information that might be relevant to the company's interests or the worker's job performance; military physicians may be expected to report a patient's infraction of the rules (such as drug use) or to assess and report on a soldier's fitness for duty.

At a minimum, the physician must ensure that patients understand the limits of confidentiality in these contexts. As employees, physicians should strive to clarify their medical care responsibilities, with the goal of identifying and avoiding circumstances that would compromise professional ethics.

That being said, employed physicians may still find themselves, like Dr. Gorden in this case, being asked or ordered to do things that run counter to their professional ethics. Employed physicians must work within their institutions to ensure that their concerns, and those of their patients, are heard and respected. The physician should remain a patient advocate, regardless of whether the patient is a military enlistee, HMO enrollee, industry employee, or prison inmate.

Medicalization of the Death Penalty

Execution by lethal doses of drugs is the most popular method of carrying out the death penalty in the United States. It is considered the most humane method of killing, and it is effective and relatively inexpensive. Physicians, who have traditionally been expected in execution chambers even before there were lethal injections, risk even greater involvement because this method is an application of medical skills and technology.

Historically, physician participation in executions has occurred because of the need for special medical skills. Regulations often require physician attendance at electrocution and poisonous gas executions to pronounce the cessation of vital signs. Doctors are also called upon to determine if a condemned person is competent to comprehend his or her fate. Lethal injection execution might then be viewed as another step in the progression of medical involvement in executions.

The profession of medicine must analyze its ability to separate itself from lethal injection executions even though ethical proscriptions exist. Physicians possess technical expertise to carry out the procedure and are likely to be consulted regarding drugs and devices. Even if physicians do not perform the lethal injection execution, the medical profession may appear involved because the method is a medical procedure.

In the present case, it would be unethical for Dr. Gorden to comply with the warden's request to participate. But even if Dr. Gorden refuses, there may be the appearance that the profession is involved. It is not surprising that the warden's response to a problem is carrying out a "medical task" (placing an intravenous catheter) is to call the doctor. Inmates and the public may have the same perception.

The medical profession itself may need to evaluate the purposes to which its technology and even its image are applied in the case of lethal injection executions. And as this method becomes increasingly commonplace in the United States, the medical profession must clearly distinguish itself from the process of lethal injection executions. The profession should be prepared to support individual physicians who uphold the ethical proscription and to sanction those who do not. Yet, it may be that much of the political acceptability of lethal injection executions stems from the perception that the procedure is a medical one, and that the medical profession is committed to humanity and relief of suffering. The profession must guard against any political distortion of its public trust.

A similar version of this case study was originally published in ACP Observer in January 1993.

REFERENCES

1. American College of Physicians. Ethics Manual, 3rd ed. Ann Intern Med. 1992; 117:947-60.
2. American College of Physicians. Defining Physician Participation in State Executions. American Medical Association Resolution 5, Interim Meeting 1991.

ANNOTATED BIBLIOGRAPHY

Farber N, Davis EB, Weiner J, et al. Physicians' attitudes about involvement in lethal injection for capital punishment. Arch Intern Med. 2000;160:2912-6.

A survey that assesses how physicians feel about a potential role in the process of capital punishment, specifically in certain actions allowed and disallowed by the American Medical Association.

Emanuel LL, Bienen LB. Physician participation in executions: time to eliminate anonymity provisions and protest the practice. Ann Intern Med. 2001;135:922-4.

The authors believe that doctors need to be aware of their fiduciary responsibility to patients. The paper also addresses the study of physician involvement in lethal injections conducted by Farber et al (above) and claims that the willing doctor participants are a "confused minority."

Sikora A, Flieschman AR. Physician participation in capital punishment: a question of professional integrity. J Urban Health. 1999;76:400-40.

Authors argue that it is unethical for medical professionals to participate in capital punishment and that a severe consequence of participation is the erosion of trust in the practice of medicine.

Ragon SA. A doctor's dilemma: resolving the conflict between physician participation in executions and the AMA's Code of Medical Ethics. University of Dayton Law Review. 1995;20:957-1007.

Examines the issue of physician involvement in capital punishment and conflicts between American Medical Association guidelines and state laws. Attempts to find potential resolutions to this ethical dilemma but concludes that doctors should be removed from the execution process and that other, non-medical, personnel should be trained for the role.

21

Ethics and Medicaid Patients

Commentary by Lois Snyder, JD
Case History by Janet Weiner, MPH, and Lois Snyder, JD

Case History

Harvey Mitchell is an internist in solo practice in a small city in the Northeast. One day he receives a message to call an old classmate, Linda Cohen, who practices in an academic medical center at the other end of the state. The message indicates that Dr. Cohen would like to refer a patient named Bernadine Johnson, who is moving to Dr. Mitchell's area. Dr. Mitchell returns the call the following day, only to discover that Dr. Cohen is out of town. He tells Dr. Cohen's secretary that he would be happy to see Ms. Johnson and to ask the patient to authorize the transfer of records. Dr. Mitchell tells his receptionist to schedule Ms. Johnson if she calls and also mentions it to his nurse, who often screens new patients over the phone to assess their needs.

A few days later, Dr. Mitchell's nurse buzzes his office. She says, "You remember that referral from Dr. Cohen you mentioned? Well, she just called for an appointment, and I said I'd get back to her. She has Medicaid, and it took me 20 minutes just to review all of her problems on the phone. In case you didn't know . . . She has poorly controlled diabetes with congestive heart failure, a chronic non-healing foot ulcer, peripheral neuropathy, retinopathy, and recurrent urinary tract infections. She wants us to coordinate all her care and to make appointments with the specialists she needs. What do you want me to do?" Dr. Mitchell sighs and says, "Tell her that we're not taking any new patients and give her Dr. Perry's number."

The following day, Dr. Cohen calls Dr. Mitchell. "Harvey, I just heard from Bernadine Johnson, who said she couldn't get an

continued on page 131

Case History *continued from page 130*

appointment at your office. Did your receptionist make a mistake?" Dr. Mitchell hedges. "Well, it's been really busy here. Besides, it sounds as though she would be better off with Dr. Perry, who works in the community health center."

"But, Harvey, I referred her to you because her care is complex and I trust your judgment as a physician. Do you only see a certain kind of patient? Why are you turning her away?" Dr. Cohen asks, her anger rising. "How can you justify discrimination?"

Dr. Mitchell remains calm. "This isn't about discrimination. It's that I just can't accept Medicaid patients. Look, don't judge me—I'm out here in private practice, and I lose money on every Medicaid patient, not to mention one with this many problems. Even if I see her, there's no way I can get her the consults she needs. Do you know how much Medicaid pays for an initial visit? You may not have to face economic realities in your situation, but I can't avoid them in mine."

Is Dr. Mitchell ethically justified in refusing to care for Ms. Johnson?

Commentary

But in truth, one ought always to ask oneself what would happen if everyone did as one is doing. —Jean-Paul Sartre

The initiation of the patient-physician relationship is based on mutual agreement regarding medical care for the patient. A physician may not discriminate against a class or category of patients who fall within his or her specialty; however, as stated in the American College of Physicians (ACP) Ethics Manual, in the absence of an existing relationship, a physician is not ethically obligated to provide care to an individual except in specific situations, such as an emergency, under a contract, or when no other physician is available (1).

In this case, if Dr. Mitchell refused to care for all patients of a particular race, the case would be a clear one of unethical discrimination against a class. If he refused to care for a patient of that race because he knew from another physician, for example, of that patient's history of prescription drug fraud activities, the case would also be clear: no ethical obligation. But Dr. Mitchell says he cannot accept Ms. Johnson as a patient because she has Medicaid.

Clearly, Dr. Mitchell is not ethically obligated to accept all Medicaid patients into his practice. The context for deciding to accept any individual patient, i.e., the current composition of a practice, is an important factor. Dr. Mitchell might already have many Medicaid patients, or he might be a regular volunteer at the free clinic. Also important is the selection process. Is it ethical for a physician to regularly use criteria other than clinical expertise and factors intrinsic to the patient-physician relationship in choosing patients? Would Dr. Mitchell be on the same moral footing when he refuses new patients because their illness is not within his area of competence, because he does not speak their language, or because the patients do not have private insurance?

The ACP Ethics Manual states unequivocally that the welfare of the patient must take primacy over the physician's fiscal considerations. The Ethics Manual is less clear, however, on the role of fiscal considerations in the physician's acceptance of a new patient.

In 1990, Medicaid reimbursement levels averaged 69% of Medicare prevailing charges and an even lesser percentage of private insurance payments (2). It is conceivable that a private practice could not be sustained on Medicaid reimbursement alone. Dr. Mitchell's decision is certainly ethical if accepting Medicaid threatens the viability of his practice (in which case all his patients will suffer). Ethics does not require that he accept all people who have Medicaid any more than he is required to work 18 hours a day in order to meet the needs of all potential patients. But does that mean he is ethically justified if he does not accept any Medicaid patients?

When Dr. Mitchell says, "I lose money on every Medicaid patient," he probably means that Medicaid reimbursement does not cover his overhead costs, averaged out for each patient. But general internists see an average of 117 patients per week, and the vast majority of those patients do not have Medicaid (3). If Dr. Mitchell's practice is typical, the marginal cost of a few Medicaid patients would not threaten his practice or dramatically lower his overall income level. The key lies in a fair and equitable distribution of Medicaid patients throughout medical practices. Physicians can satisfy both ethical and financial requirements by a commitment to this fair-share principle.

However, a 1992 report by the American Medical Association's Council on Ethical and Judicial Affairs stated that as many as one-third of physicians provided little or no free or reduced-pay care and that "a disproportionate share of uncompensated care was provided by those practices which already had relatively high levels of Medicaid patients" (4). Some physicians are not seeing their fair share of the less-profitable patients. If other physicians in the community are willing to accept Medicaid patients, are the physicians who do not accept them relieved of their obligation? How many physicians are referring to Dr. Perry at the community health center? Is it fair to their colleagues for some physicians to avoid the less financially appealing patients, especially those needing complex care? Is it fair to the patients who get left out? Does this satisfy the collective obligation of the medical profession to society?

Some physicians might avoid this obligation because they believe that Medicaid patients are more likely to sue or that their presence in the waiting room will cause non-Medicaid patients to leave (5,6). However, recent studies comparing medical malpractice claims by Medicaid vs. non-Medicaid recipients do not support the belief that Medicaid patients are more litigious (6,7). One physician whose practice includes a large number of Medicaid patients had this to say about his mix of patients: "Although many colleagues tell me off the record that they shun Medicaid chiefly out of fear of losing private patients, I've found such defections to be largely a myth. Currently, about half my patients are Medicaid recipients, yet I've heard no complaints from the non-Medicaid segment" (5).

Although they are a fact of life, financial considerations should not interfere with the physician's primary commitment to patients. Reform that replaces our current patchwork approach to health care with a cohesive and coherent system that provides adequate access to care for all Americans is much needed. Reimbursement is most properly dealt with as a policy matter at the system level, not at the level of physician and patient.

As a practical matter, any given patient will probably ultimately receive care, albeit perhaps after being shuffled from physician to physician or to a clinic. Or the patient might end up in the emergency room. But delaying care can hurt patients and be inefficient. To enter the medical profession is to recognize the obligation to participate in medicine's collective responsibility to all who are sick, and to ensure that resources are used wisely. Otherwise the profession has a collective duty that no one physician is obligated to fulfill. Where once the profession taught its students and young physicians the "ancient message that a physician is bound by 'professing' humane kindness (*humanitas*) and compassion (*misericordia*) to those in need," one physician has noted that any sense of obligation to care for the poor is diminishing and that, as a consequence, the cynicism of both physicians and patients is fueled when young physicians are taught that they may put their own financial interests ahead of patient needs (8).

This cynicism is fueled further by the reluctance on the part of some physicians to be honest about their reasons for refusing patients. As in this case, if a "wrong" answer is given to an appointment secretary's inquiry about insurance or ability to pay, there can suddenly be no room in the doctor's schedule for a new patient. This phenomenon has been written about as it applies to Medicare patients (9). Obviously, lying to a prospective patient or the referring physician about the reason for not accepting the individual cannot be condoned. Truth-telling is a basic tenet of the medical profession; it is essential to relationships with colleagues and patients, and the social contract within which medicine is practiced.

Every physician should participate in implementing the fair-share principle. This can be done by providing care to the poor in the office setting at no cost or at reduced cost, by serving at clinics that treat the poor or shelters for the homeless or abused women, by accepting Medicaid patients in sufficient numbers, or by participating in programs developed by medical societies to care for those in need.

How much is fair? The American Medical Association's Council on Ethical and Judicial Affairs has said:

"The measure of what constitutes an appropriate contribution may vary with circumstances such as community characteristics, geographic location, the nature of the physician's practice and specialty, and other conditions. All physicians should work to ensure that the needs of the poor in their communities are met. Caring for the poor should become a normal part of the physician's overall service to patients.

"In the poorest communities, it may not be possible to meet the needs of the indigent for physicians' services by relying solely on local physicians. The local physicians should be able to turn for assistance to their colleagues in prosperous communities, particularly those in close proximity.

"State, local, and specialty medical societies should help physicians meet their obligations to provide care to the indigent" (4).

Dr. Mitchell might have decided long ago that he will not accept any Medicaid patients. Or he may have a waiting room with many Medicaid patients and merely be refusing to accept another. However, based on a fair-share principle, the latter explanation seems ethically defensible whereas the former does not.

A similar version of this case study was originally published in ACP Observer in March 1993.

REFERENCES

1. American College of Physicians. Ethics Manual, 3rd ed. Ann Intern Med. 1992; 117:947-60.
2. Physician Payment Review Commission. Annual Report to Congress 1991. Washington, DC; 1991.
3. American Medical Association. Physician Marketplace Statistics 1991. Chicago, 1991.
4. The Council on Ethical and Judicial Affairs of the American Medical Association. AMA Council Report C: Caring for the Poor (1992).
5. Attwood C. It's unfair—and unwise—to shun Medicaid patients. Medical Economics. 1991;22-8.

6. McNulty M. Questions and answers: are poor patients likely to sue for malpractice? JAMA. 1989;262:1391-2.
7. Mussman MG, Zawistowich L, Weisman CS, et al. Medical malpractice claims filed by Medicaid and non-Medicaid recipients in Maryland. JAMA. 1991;265:2992-4.
8. Miles SH. What are we teaching about indigent patients? JAMA. 1992;268:2562-3.
9. Butler RN. Doctors are refusing to treat Medicare patients. The Washington Post. 12 May 1992.

ANNOTATED BIBLIOGRAPHY

Caring for the poor. JAMA. 1993;269:2533-7.

The AMA looks at how the poor were historically cared for, identifies current problems, and finds that every physician has a duty to share in providing care to the indigent and that medical societies should assist physicians in meeting this responsibility.

Gordon HL, Reiser SJ. Do physicians have a duty to treat Medicare patients? Arch Intern Med. 1993;153:563-5.

Examines arguments for and against accepting Medicare patients and asserts that all doctors should serve the patient, including Medicare patients, but also calls for changes in Medicare to ease economic and administrative barriers to care.

Miles SH. What are we teaching about indigent patients? JAMA. 1992;268:2562-3.

Uses a case to explore physician obligations and the message being sent to physicians in training when hospitals transfer patients based on their inability to pay. Finds that fiscal limits on patient care go beyond simple practice environment issues to pose basic ethical questions and choices for medicine as a profession. An eloquent call to arms.

22

The Duty to Treat HIV-Positive Patients
Commentary and Case History by Janet Weiner, MPH

Case History

John Alden, 40, has chronic stable angina that does not respond to medical therapies. He makes a return visit to Dr. Standish, an internist who has followed him for 5 years. In taking the interval history, Dr. Standish finds that Mr. Alden had HIV testing a year ago at an anonymous site and is HIV-positive. Mr. Alden reports that he feels well in general but has noticed significant worsening of his chest pain. His physical examination is unchanged. Because of the change in Mr. Alden's cardiac symptoms, Dr. Standish orders an exercise thallium scan, which suggests two-vessel involvement.

Dr. Standish refers Mr. Alden to Dr. Montgomery, head of cardiology at Sheridan Hospital, for a same-day catheterization. Dr. Montgomery, in reviewing the medical records, notes that Mr. Alden is HIV-positive. He states that he and his staff have decided to refuse to perform elective cardiac catherization on HIV-positive patients. Dr. Standish is shocked and accuses Dr. Montgomery of gross dereliction of his duty to patients.

Dr. Montgomery is offended. He claims the risk of HIV transmission to his staff far outweighs the benefits for the patient, especially in the long term. He explains that this decision was not made lightly; it was in response to the recent discovery that his chief resident seroconverted after exposure to the virus during a procedure. Subsequently, the entire medical staff petitioned the hospital to test all patients for HIV on admission. The request was denied because of legal concerns and inadequate counseling services for HIV-positive patients.

Furthermore, Dr. Montgomery continues, the medical staff strongly believes that universal precautions do not adequately pro-

continued on page 137

Case History *continued from page 136*

tect physicians doing invasive procedures. Additionally, the house staff has no life or disability insurance in the event of HIV infection. Because the hospital is in an area of high HIV prevalence, the staff deemed these risks unacceptably high. Dr. Montgomery says that the hospital administration, while not fully agreeing with this position, supports the staff's decision. He believes Mr. Alden's best interests would be served by referring him to another cardiac care center.

On hearing all of this, Dr. Standish is somewhat sympathetic but fails to be persuaded. He will not be able to follow Mr. Alden through his catheterization, possible surgery, and recovery at another hospital at which he does not have privileges. He does not know what to tell to Mr. Alden, and wonders what this experience tells him about voluntary HIV testing.

Commentary

The American College of Physicians, among other groups, has upheld the physician's "duty to treat" AIDS and HIV-positive patients, drawing upon the professionalism of medicine. "It is inappropriate for any health care professional to compromise the treatment of any patient, including those with transmissible, lethal diseases such as AIDS, on the grounds that such patients present unacceptable medical risks" (1). The American College of Physicians Ethics Manual states that "a physician may not discriminate against a class or category of patients . . ." (2).

This case study illustrates the difficulties and conflicts physicians may face in fulfilling their obligations to patients. In practical terms, no obligation is absolute. What are the boundaries of this duty to treat, and how can ethical parameters guide individual physicians in the wake of AIDS?

The ethical imperative to treat AIDS patients stems from the duty to treat all classes of patients within a physician's sphere of competence. While a physician is not obligated to treat any one patient (except in certain circumstances, such as in an emergency room or on call), refusing to treat entire groups of people violates the values of professional responsibility.

Contrast this with a more commercial model of physician responsibility, in which physicians are not obligated to treat any person or group. In this model, medicine is more like a trade: physicians are business people who sell their skills to consumers (patients), and become obligated only through contractual arrangements (3).

The American College of Physicians has consistently rejected this as the sole interpretation of the physician-patient relationship. "The practice of medicine is a societal trust and carries with it a societal responsibility. If medicine wishes to retain its respected status as the healing profession, we must continue to provide the best possible care to our patients, regardless of risk" (1).

Assuming that the physicians in this example accept this notion of professional responsibility, how can we understand their different positions? Dr. Standish wants to provide the best care he can to Mr. Alden by referring him appropriately and following him through the length of his hospital stay and recovery. He believes that Mr. Alden's HIV status does not preclude an elective workup of angina because he is asymptomatic for HIV infection, and he is likely to live many years. As a general internist, Dr. Standish does not do invasive procedures and believes universal precautions adequately protect him from HIV infection.

Dr. Montgomery, on the other hand, runs the cardiac catheterization laboratory, where parenteral blood exposures occur frequently. One staff member has already seroconverted, and Dr. Montgomery has heard estimates of a 0.5% to 12% annual risk of infection for surgeons and other physicians doing invasive procedures in high-prevalence areas (4,5). He believes that the cumulative risk of death is unacceptable for his staff, especially when weighed against the marginal benefits to many HIV-positive patients.

However, recent data do not support the magnitude of risk that Dr. Montgomery presupposes. The cumulative risk for HIV infection in health care workers depends on three variables: the prevalence of the virus in the patient population, the frequency of needlestick exposures, and the risk of seroconversion from a single contaminated needlestick (5).

In a study of surgical personnel at the San Francisco General Hospital, Gerberding and colleagues calculate a theoretical risk for occupational HIV infection of 0.125 infections per year, or one infection among surgical personnel every 8 years (6). As the authors state, even this level of risk represents a major life-threatening occupational hazard for surgical personnel at San Francisco General. In places of average (less than 3%) HIV prevalence, the risk would be reduced to one infection in the surgical staff every 80 years.

Dr. Montgomery also confuses the equation in medical decision-making by weighing the risks to the physician against the benefits to the patient. Clinical indications consist of the patient's risks and benefits: although an elective cardiac workup may not be indicated for an acutely ill AIDS patient, that decision is based on medical futility (itself a complex, controversial issue). Dr. Montgomery would have to prove that the prognosis for Mr. Alden makes the workup futile, an untenable position these days.

Nevertheless, Dr. Montgomery does have a moral responsibility to minimize risk to his staff. He is on more solid ethical footing if the results of routine HIV testing are used to manage risk without compromising patient care. This is true only if evidence indicates physician knowledge of the patient's HIV status reduces risk to the medical staff, and if all patients give truly informed consent. There is some evidence against the first point; in fact, some commentators have suggested that HIV testing of patients will put physicians at greater risk because they will be reassured by negative results, some of which will be false.

Lastly, Dr. Montgomery believes that the current climate of fear and hesitation at Sheridan Hospital, given the chief resident's seroconversion, precludes providing optimal care to Mr. Alden. Because there are a number of other cardiac care centers nearby, he does not feel that he has abrogated his professional responsibility to patients but has achieved a delicate balance between his "duty to treat" and his moral obligation to his staff.

Dr. Standish cannot agree. While he acknowledges that Mr. Alden can get good care at another hospital, he does not believe that the staff at Sheridan Hospital has fulfilled its duties. He recognizes that referring his patient elsewhere may be the best compromise in this instance. But his patient may suffer from the discontinuity of care and spend more time and money traveling to another center. Dr. Standish is also concerned about the staff's categorical refusal to treat HIV-positive patients. How can medicine, as a profession, meet its collective obligation to patients if all physicians do not share the burden?

The "duty to treat" has little meaning if fear or inexperience excuses physicians from their responsibilities. It is disingenuous, and somewhat circular, for a physician to claim that fear of a class of patients precludes optimal care and justifies refusing to treat the entire class. Fear and deliberate inexperience can interfere with patient care, but physicians have a moral responsibility to confront and overcome personal barriers, rather than just referring patients to other physicians.

In turn, medical institutions have a responsibility to minimize the actual and perceived risk to their medical staffs. As one HIV-positive resident wrote, "A safe work environment also means one in which health workers are well protected economically, with appropriate health, disability, and life insurance" (7). Sheridan Hospital might arrange lectures and discussions about HIV and its transmission; train the staff in universal precautions and stress strict adherence to them; invite the staff to suggest further precautions that might enhance safety without compromising patient care; and review life and disability coverage to ensure adequate financial protection for the entire staff.

Finally, after confronting fear and overcoming inexperience, physicians must grapple with the bounds of acceptable risk. Some risks are too great even for dedicated professionals. Soldiers are not duty-bound to perform suicide missions nor are firefighters required to enter buildings on the verge of collapse (5). The occupational risk of HIV transmission should be judged relative to risks faced by other professionals and to other risks faced by physicians.

Conflicts surrounding hazardous duty have existed as long as the medical profession itself; history reveals that physicians struggled with ethical conduct in the face of epidemics such as bubonic plague, yellow fever, smallpox, and cholera, often surrounded by large and largely unexplored risks to their lives (8). Some physicians fled or refused to treat the victims; others cared selflessly for all the sick, and some died with their patients.

So, although occupational risk is not new to physicians, AIDS has introduced the problem to generations of physicians relatively unaccustomed to confronting real personal danger as they deliver medical care. The stigma of the diagnosis, the devastation of the illness itself, and the persistent media attention have combined to highlight this occupational risk above all others.

In fact, physicians are at far greater risk for hepatitis B and tuberculosis infection than HIV infection. An estimated 12,000 health care workers become infected yearly with the hepatitis B virus (HBV), and 250 eventually die from it (9). Of all health care workers, 15%-30% show evidence of exposure to HBV, which is far more infectious than HIV. The risk of HIV infection after needle-stick exposure to contaminated blood is 0.5%, compared with 6%-30% for HBV. Despite the availability of a fairly effective vaccine, many physicians do not protect themselves against HBV infection (10). Clearly, physicians accept this level of occupational risk, and refusing to treat HIV-positive patients must be viewed in this context. AIDS has provoked a degree of fear unparalleled in recent memory, a fear to which physicians are not immune.

In a national survey, 75% of 2450 physician respondents agreed with the following statement: "A physician may not ethically refuse to treat a patient whose condition is within the physician's current realm of competence solely because the patient is seropositive (for HIV)" (11). However, there were statistically significant differences among and within specialties. General internists (85%) were more likely than internal medicine subspecialists (73%) to agree with the statement. While the precise reasons for this pattern are unclear, the authors noted that many medical subspecialists perform procedures that may increase their perceived risk. General surgeons (69%), surgical specialists (59%), and obstetricians/gynecologists (64%) were less likely to feel that physicians have an ethical responsibility to treat HIV-positive patients.

AIDS offers us a critical test of the ethical parameters of the duty to treat, as well as an opportunity to reaffirm medical values and principles. By societal and professional standards, the American College of Physicians reaffirms the ethical imperative to deliver quality care to HIV-positive and AIDS patients.

A similar version of this case study was originally published in ACP Observer in February 1991.

REFERENCES

1. American College of Physicians and the Infectious Disease Society of America. The acquired immunodeficiency syndrome (AIDS) and infection with the human immunodeficiency virus (HIV). Ann Intern Med. 1988;108:460-9.
2. American College of Physicians. Ethics Manual, 2nd ed, Part 1. Ann Intern Med. 1989;111:245-52.
3. Annas GJ. Not saints, but healers: the legal duties of health care professionals in the AIDS epidemic. Am J Pub Health. 1988;78:844-9.
4. Task Force on AIDS and Orthopedic Surgery. Recommendations for the Prevention of Human Immunodeficiency Virus (HIV) Transmission in the Practice of Orthopedic Surgery. American Academy of Orthopedic Surgeons, July 1989.
5. Emanuel EJ. Do physicians have an obligation to treat patients with AIDS? N Engl J Med. 1988;318:1686-90.
6. Gerberding JL, Littell C, Tarkington A, et al. Risk of exposure of surgical personnel to patients' blood during surgery at San Francisco General Hospital. N Engl J Med. 1990;322:1788-93.
7. Aoun H. When a house officer gets AIDS. N Engl J Med. 1989;321:693-6.
8. Zuger A, Miles SH. AIDS and occupational risk: historic traditions and ethical obligations. JAMA. 1987;258:1924-8.
9. Centers for Disease Control. Guidelines for the prevention of transmission of human immunodeficiency virus and hepatitis B virus to health-care and public-safety workers. MMWR. 1989;38:S-6.
10. ACP Task Force on Adult Immunization and Infectious Diseases Society of America. Guide for Adult Immunization, 2nd ed. Philadelphia: American College of Physicians; 1990.
11. Rizzo JA, Marder WD, Willke RJ. Physician contact with and attitudes toward HIV-seropositive patients: results from a national survey. Med Care. 1990;28:251-60.

ANNOTATED BIBLIOGRAPHY

Annas GJ. Not saints, but healers: the legal duties of health care professionals in the AIDS epidemic. Am J Pub Health. 1988;78:844-9.

Reviews legal history and thought and provides a framework for encouraging the duty to treat as a matter of ethics.

Cooke M. Patient rights and physician responsibility: four problems in AIDS care. In: Volberding P, Jacobson MA, eds. AIDS Clinical Review 1993/1994. New York: Marcel Dekker; 1994.

Encourages expansion of the number of providers willing to treat HIV-infected patients under a section on the right to receive care. Also includes sections on the right to control the medical record, the right to experimental therapies, and the right to die.

Emanuel EJ. Do physicians have an obligation to treat patients with AIDS? N Engl J Med. 1988;318:1686-90.

Although this responsibility can be tempered by factors such as excessive risk, the author argues that individual physicians have this obligation as members of a learned profession who care for the ill.

Gerbert BG, Maguire BT, Bleecker T, et al. Primary care physicians and AIDS: attitudinal and structural barriers to care. JAMA. 1991;266:2837-42.

This survey found that most primary care physicians believed in a duty to treat HIV-infected patients but also found obstacles to care, such as negativity toward certain patient groups, and time constraints that limit care.

Zuger A, Miles SH. Physicians, AIDS, and occupational risk: historic traditions and ethical obligations. JAMA. 1987;258:1924-8.

Examines physician responses to other deadly contagious diseases and affirms a duty to treat AIDS based on medicine as moral enterprise.

23

The Impaired Colleague

Commentary by Janet Weiner, MPH, and Lois Snyder, JD
Case History by Janet Weiner, MPH

Case History

Paul Daniels is an associate professor of medicine at General Hospital. He is well known for his clinical and diagnostic skills, and sees many patients who are referred to him because their cases are clinical "puzzles." He has been at General Hospital for 10 years, through internship and residency, and is respected within the institution.

Carla Martin is a recently appointed assistant professor of medicine at General Hospital. At a Saturday faculty party, Dr. Martin notices Dr. Daniels slurring his words and staggering; she is concerned about Dr. Daniels driving home while intoxicated. He assures her that he is sober and can drive safely.

During this conversation, Dr. Daniels' beeper goes off, and he answers his page. Dr. Martin overhears the discussion between Dr. Daniels and a new intern, and realizes that Dr. Daniels is on call. She hears Dr. Daniels prescribe an unusually large dose of digoxin for the patient in question. When Dr. Martin asks Dr. Daniels about the patient, he says the problem was routine and that the new intern had July-itis.

Dr. Martin worries all weekend about the patient on digoxin. On Monday morning, she finds the patient and reviews the chart. The intern had not followed Dr. Daniels' instructions but had given the patient a much lower dose. Dr. Martin tracks down the intern and asks about the digoxin dosage. The intern says that she checked with a more senior resident because she thought she misheard Dr. Daniels' directions and that she had given the lower dosage upon the resident's instructions. Dr. Martin assures the apologetic

continued on page 144

Case History *continued from page 143*

intern that she gave the patient the correct dosage but does not tell her about Dr. Daniels' mistake.

That day, Dr. Martin tries to discuss the issue with Dr. Daniels, who tells her that she is completely out of line. He denies any inappropriate behavior or having a drinking problem. He questions Dr. Martin's motives and tells her to mind her own business.

Dr. Martin makes discreet inquiries about Dr. Daniels and discovers that other faculty members have noticed him drinking excessively at parties. In fact, his friends on the staff often draw straws to decide who will drive him home after a party. No one seems to be concerned about Dr. Daniels' clinical competence. As Dr. Martin decides what to do, she looks into programs at General Hospital for employees with substance abuse problems. She finds that General Hospital has had a voluntary, confidential program in place for 10 years. When a physician is involved, an immediate assessment is made of the physician's clinical competence and threat to patient safety. Clinical performance is monitored directly.

Dr. Martin is unsure about her next steps. Being relatively new to General Hospital, she questions her interpretation of Dr. Daniels' behavior. Other faculty members who have known Dr. Daniels for a long time, seem unconcerned about his drinking. What should she do?

Commentary

This case study highlights the difficult issues surrounding the professional mandate to protect patients from physicians impaired by psychiatric, physiological, or physical disorders. The American College of Physicians Ethics Manual is unequivocal: "It is the responsibility of every physician to protect the public from an impaired physician . . . All steps must be taken to ensure that no patient is harmed because of actions or decisions made by an impaired physician" (1). But upholding this duty often necessitates making a judgment about a colleague's impairment, as well as confronting institutional, social, and personal barriers.

In this case study, Dr. Martin has direct evidence that a patient could have been harmed by Dr. Daniels' actions. Although she might not be in the best position to judge the level of his impairment because she has limited experience with Dr. Daniels and is new to the institution, she has a moral duty to ensure that his impairment and clinical competence are assessed by an appropriate authority.

Dr. Daniels should be confronted again and told to seek help, particularly through General Hospital's voluntary, confidential program. Dr. Martin could try this or inform the appropriate parties within the institution (possibly the division or department chief) about the incident she witnessed and her conversation with the young intern. If the institutional authorities fail to act, Dr. Martin should consider reporting Dr. Daniels to the state medical society (most societies have impaired physician programs).

We can envision the dilemmas facing Dr. Martin as she tries to fulfill her obligations. In General Hospital, Dr. Daniels is respected, well-known, and tenured. Dr. Martin is a relatively new faculty member whose future at the hospital could be at stake. She might also have a normal aversion to confrontation, especially about a topic as sensitive as physician impairment. She might worry about losing the respect and trust of her peers, and about the legal implications of making such an accusation. Clearly, Dr. Martin takes a certain risk, personally and professionally, by pursuing this issue.

However, confronting Dr. Daniels, or reporting him, need not be seen exclusively in a negative light. Great progress has been made in the treatment of the impaired physician in the past 20 years, since the American Medical Association produced its landmark report, "The Sick Physician." In 1973 it adopted the program recommended in its report, which stressed the physician's ethical obligation to help impaired colleagues while ensuring that impaired physicians do not endanger patients (2). Most programs now emphasize treatment and rehabilitation, rather than discipline and sanctions. And recovery rates for physicians are higher than the general population: in a case control study, 83% of physicians had returned to practice and were functioning well 3 years after treatment, compared with 62% of non-physician middle-class control subjects (2).

Dr. Martin may also worry about her legal duties and protection. While statutes vary from state to state, many states have instituted "snitch laws" that require certain groups of people (such as physician colleagues and health care entities) to report knowledge of physician impairment to either a state medical society or licensing board (3).

Most laws provide a certain degree of anonymity for reporting parties as well as immunity from a civil suit, while setting penalties for those designated who do not report an impaired physician. Most laws also allow the impaired physician's records to remain confidential. Dr. Martin should contact her state medical society to find out the legal requirements in her state.

Regardless of Dr. Martin's legal duties, she is morally required to protect patients from harm. She must resist a natural impulse to not get involved, especially given that this colleague is a senior one, or to identify with Dr. Daniels (there but for the grace of God . . .). Certainly, she should act carefully and discreetly, but she must also take definitive action.

How far does Dr. Martin's obligation extend? If Dr. Daniels agrees to seek treatment, how can Dr. Martin be sure he goes? Is it even appropriate for her to check? If she reports Dr. Daniels to the department head, is her obligation fulfilled even if the department head fails to act? In other words, when has Dr. Martin done enough?

We do not see easy answers to these questions. There may be limits to what Dr. Martin can do within her institution and in her role as Dr. Daniels' colleague. One person cannot become completely responsible for the actions of another. However, it is reasonable to use the following rule as a guide: A physician's obligation corresponds to how much evidence exists that a patient could be harmed.

In our case study, Dr. Martin knows that a patient could have been harmed, and she should assume that Dr. Daniels' other patients are at risk. Thus, her obligation extends further than if she had only noticed Dr. Daniels drinking excessively at a party when he was not on call. In that case, it might have been sufficient to express her concern to Dr. Daniels only, and to remain alert to other signs of Dr. Daniels' potential impairment.

While we have emphasized Dr. Martin's ethical obligations here, we do not minimize Dr. Daniels' responsibility for his own behavior. He clearly violated the maxim *Primum non nocere* ("First, do no harm"), which has been a cornerstone of physician ethics for centuries.

Beyond the direct threat to patient safety, Dr. Daniels' drinking could also have dire consequences for the young interns and residents he supervises.

Clearly, Dr. Daniels bears the ultimate responsibility for his impairment. But this acknowledgment should not obscure the nature of Dr. Daniels' problem, which is substance abuse. At every step, the ultimate goal of all parties (the impaired physician, knowing colleagues, and the institution itself) is the protection of patients, followed by the rehabilitation of the impaired physician and a return to clinical competence.

A similar version of this case study was originally published in ACP Observer in September 1991.

REFERENCES

1. American College of Physicians. Ethics Manual, 2nd ed, Part 1: History, the patient, other physicians. Ann Intern Med. 1989;111:254-2; Part 2: The physician and society. Research: Life-sustaining treatment; Other issues. Ann Intern Med. 1989;111:327-35.
2. Sargent DA. The impaired physician movement: an interim report. Hosp Comm Psychiatry. 1985;36:294-7.
3. Walzer RS. Impaired physicians: an overview and update of the legal issues. J Leg Med. 1990;11:131-98.

ANNOTATED BIBLIOGRAPHY

Boisaubin EV, Levine RE. Identifying and assisting the impaired physician. Am J Med Sci. 2001;322:31-6.

Defines physician impairment and factors in its development, estimating that about 15% of physicians will be impaired at some point in their careers. Stresses identification of impaired clinicians as essential because patient well-being may be at stake and untreated impairment may result in loss of license and further health problems for the impaired individual. Reviews physician recovery experience.

Centrella M. Physician addiction and impairment. Current thinking: a review. J Addictive Dis. 1994;13:91-105.

Looks at definitions, prevalence, diagnosis, treatment, rehabilitation, prevention, and other aspects of physician impairment with an emphasis on what works.

Deckard G, Meterko M, Field D. Physician burnout: an examination of personal, professional, and organizational relationships. Medical Care. 1994;32:745-54.

Three PhDs empirically assess burnout among staff model HMO doctors and recommend that organizations review policies, procedures, and management structures that contribute to high rates of emotional exhaustion and other manifestations of burnout.

Morreim H. Am I my brother's warden? Responding to the unethical or incompetent colleague. Hastings Center Rep. 1993;23:19-27.

Physicians must care for their own and respond to unethical or incompetent colleagues lest the integrity of the entire profession be compromised. Points out the incentives to not get involved, but exhorts that physicians must take responsibility for self-regulation.

Reid WH. Recognizing and dealing with impaired clinicians, Part 1: Recognition and reporting. J Med Pract Manage. 2001;17:97-9.

Failure to report impaired or incompetent physicians can harm patients, the profession, and the clinician. This article discusses how to recognize and handle impaired clinicians.

24

When Residents and Attendings Disagree

Commentary and Case History by Errol D. Crook, MD, and Janet Weiner, MPH

Case History

Two months ago Mr. Jones, age 60 and a cigarette smoker, was diagnosed with unresectable squamous cell carcinoma of the lung. He had previously been in good health and had not seen a doctor in years. Unfortunately, the plant he had worked in for several years recently closed and he could not afford to continue his medical insurance.

Susan Shaw, an internal medicine resident rotating on the oncology service for 2 months, took care of Mr. Jones at the county hospital when the diagnosis was made and has since seen him twice in the oncology clinic. At these encounters, Mr. Jones rarely saw an attending physician and considered Dr. Shaw his doctor. After extensive discussion with Dr. Shaw regarding the diagnosis, Mr. Jones and his wife decided on palliative therapy as the only form of treatment, although no written advance directive was created. Because Dr. Shaw plans to become an oncologist, the attendings knew her well and agreed with her plans for Mr. Jones.

Until a week ago, Mr. Jones had been doing relatively well and had been quite active. Since that time, however, he has suffered progressive shortness of breath, malaise, and a productive cough. Tonight, after developing fever and chills, he comes to the emergency department seeking relief from his symptoms. Dr. Shaw is on call and is paged to the emergency department to evaluate Mr. Jones. She diagnoses a post-obstructive pneumonia and orders antibiotics and oxygen, which moderately relieve Mr. Jones' severe shortness of breath and hypoxemia. A few hours later she returns to check on him. He still has to work hard to breathe, despite the high concentration of oxygen being

continued on page 149

Case History continued from page 148

delivered. Recognizing that there is a strong possibility that Mr. Jones' condition could worsen over the next several hours, Dr. Shaw sits down to discuss Mr. Jones' wishes with him.

Dr. Shaw informs Mr. Jones that his illness is severe and could lead to the need for mechanical ventilation. She tells him that some forms of therapy might relieve his obstruction and improve his chances of recovery. Despite his severe illness, Mr. Jones listens attentively and understands his options. He decides that he would rather not be intubated for any reason. He also decides against any form of therapy other than antibiotics to treat his pneumonia and oxygen to relieve his dyspnea. He says that he has had a good life and has come to terms with his illness.

Dr. Shaw makes note of Mr. Jones' decision; she feels comfortable with his decision, knowing that he came to it after careful analysis of all of the information given to him. He has demonstrated sound judgment and clear reasoning. She feels confident that his decision is based on a desire to live out his life without aggressive medical care, not on external or financial considerations.

The next morning Dr. Shaw presents Mr. Jones to her attending, Barry Davis. She tells him of Mr. Jones' wish not to be intubated and to forgo any therapy other than antibiotics and oxygen. After reviewing the case and X-rays, Dr. Davis feels localized external beam radiation would relieve Mr. Jones' obstruction and that he would probably recover from his pneumonia. Given his diagnosis, he had been doing well before this acute illness, which is in his favor. Dr. Davis decides to convince Mr. Jones to try the more aggressive approach.

Drs. Davis and Shaw and Mr. Jones have a lengthy conversation about Mr. Jones' tumor and pneumonia. Mr. Jones, who is in even more respiratory distress than before, stands by his earlier decision. Dr. Davis doesn't feel comfortable with that decision and asks Dr. Shaw to call the pulmonologist and radiation oncologist to see Mr. Jones. She asks why. Dr. Davis says he feels that Mr. Jones is giving up and may be denying himself several weeks to months of life. He doesn't think the patient can make a rational decision given the severity of his acute illness, and in cases like this he would rather be aggressive. "I've seen patients change their minds as they became increasingly ill, but by then it may be too late," Dr. Davis says.

Dr. Shaw disagrees with Dr. Davis' approach. She thinks that calling in consultants is a breach of Mr. Jones' well-thought-out wishes. How should Dr. Shaw handle her disagreement with Dr. Davis' plan?

Commentary

This case raises several important issues, including the ethical responsibilities of physicians-in-training, patient advocacy, and end-of-life decision-making.

Dr. Shaw is the physician with the longest and closest relationship with the patient, who depends on her for guidance in making any medical decision. Mr. Jones considers Dr. Shaw his doctor and his biggest supporter in the medical system. The role of patient advocate, foreign to many residents, carries many serious obligations.

Dr. Shaw's dual role as the physician-in-training and patient advocate has caused personal conflict. As a resident she does not have the power to make the final decision about a patient's care. And to argue vigorously for Mr. Jones' wishes could cause problems for her because she will be applying for oncology fellowships in the near future. What are her options and obligations?

The American College of Physicians Ethics Manual states that "Residents . . . are bound by the same ethical principles as other physicians [and] should acknowledge their limitations and ask for help or supervision from the attending physician, chief of service, or consultants when concerns arise about patient care" (1). What is best for the patient must be the primary concern and the patient's wishes must be respected. Therefore, Dr. Shaw should continue discussions with the patient and her attending.

She must be sure that Mr. Jones' decision does, in fact, represent what he really wants. He has to know the risks and benefits of any possible therapy as well as the consequences of refusing therapy. To this end, the consultations requested by Dr. Davis may be beneficial—not in a persuasive manner as Dr. Davis would like, but in an educational sense. The consultants may be able to provide Mr. Jones with the most complete data available about his prognosis and options, including details Dr. Shaw may not have had. As patient advocate, Dr. Shaw must be sure that any decision Mr. Jones makes is truly an informed one.

Dr. Shaw should also discuss her concerns directly with Dr. Davis. His experience provides a unique perspective into these kinds of problems that she might find eye-opening. As an oncologist, he has to deal with end-of-life decisions frequently. It is likely that his actions are based on experiences in this kind of situation, which he has faced far more often than Dr. Shaw. Dr. Davis knows that if Mr. Jones eventually changes his mind, his chances of surviving this episode might be slimmer because of the delay in starting therapy. The Ethics Manual supports a physician's right to persuade, but not to coerce, if he or she feels it is unwise for a patient to refuse therapy: "Physicians have the obligation to ensure that the refusal is truly informed, to give a clear recommendation, and to try to persuade the patient, but ultimately they must accept the patient's decision" (1).

In addition to being educational, a discussion between both physicians would give Dr. Shaw an opportunity to relay Mr. Jones' concerns as well as her own. In turn, Dr. Davis should respect the relationship between Dr. Shaw and Mr. Jones, and should give credence to Dr. Shaw's insights. Although she has not had a long-standing relationship with the patient, the length of the relationship is not as critical as the content of their interactions.

After consultations and discussions, Dr. Davis continues to try to persuade Mr. Jones to change his mind. Dr. Shaw finds herself in an even more complicated position. Because she is the only physician with an established relationship with Mr. Jones, she must continue to act on his behalf. Using the guidelines stated above, she should seek help from her chief resident or program director. She could also consult the chief of staff or the hospital ethics committee, or bring up the issue at noon conference or morning report. Dr. Shaw's options will vary from institution to institution, and she should use tact and diplomacy in deciding whom to involve first. What is best for the patient must remain primary, although Dr. Shaw is in a vulnerable position as a resident and future oncology fellow.

Should Dr. Shaw withdraw from the case? The Ethics Manual allows for residents to withdraw from cases where there may be ethical or religious concerns after in-depth discussion with the attending physician and arrangement of alternative coverage (1). However, it would not be appropriate for Dr. Shaw to withdraw from this case, given her relationship with the patient and his family. Withdrawal may be warranted in cases where the resident has personal moral objections to therapy that the patient or family wants. For example, a resident may be opposed to withdrawing tube feeding, even if the patient and family insist upon it and others agree. In our case, Dr. Shaw has no moral conflict with the patient's wishes and should continue in her role as patient advocate.

This case also points out the distinct benefits of completing an advance directive in the outpatient setting. The Patient Self-Determination Act of 1990 requires most health care institutions to inform patients, on admission, about their right to complete an advance directive. However, this requirement is no substitute for discussions and written directives at outpatient visits before the patient is acutely ill. With "advance directives, competent patients state what treatments they would accept or decline if they lost decision-making capacity . . . patients also indicate their general goals for care" (1). Mr. Jones comes to the hospital without a formal advance directive, although he has had some limited discussions with Dr. Shaw in clinic.

Why didn't Mr. Jones complete a written advance directive before he was hospitalized? He faced several possible barriers. He didn't have a primary care physician with whom he had a long relationship. "His doctor," Dr. Shaw, met him during one hospitalization, saw him only twice in clinic, and will be on this clinical service for a short time. These same barriers contributed to the conflicts during his hospitalization. The attending physician of record has not had extensive conversations with the patient, yet bears ultimate responsibility for the treatment plan.

A written advance directive would be persuasive evidence that Mr. Jones had considered these issues before becoming acutely ill. Depending on the document and state law, it may or may not be meant to apply in this situation. It would not prevent him from changing his mind during the hospitalization, as treatment options were presented to him. And it does not mean that he refuses all treatments and medical care. In each situation, the physician needs to discuss with the patient (or a surrogate, if the patient is incompetent) specific treatments, whether they are palliative, curative, or resuscitative in nature. However, having an advance directive generally indicates that the patient has given thought to some of the circumstances that might arise.

In summary, Dr. Shaw should explore several options in order to resolve her problem. She must be sure that Mr. Jones is well-informed and consistent in his decision. She may need further guidance from a chief resident or program officer but should express her concerns directly to Dr. Davis. Her primary obligation is to the patient, who considers her his strongest advocate. If Mr. Jones continues to decline further treatment, his comfort should be assured and his wishes respected.

A similar version of this case study was originally published in ACP Observer in February 1994.

REFERENCE

1. American College of Physicians. Ethics Manual, 3rd ed. Ann Intern Med. 1992; 117:947-60.

ANNOTATED BIBLIOGRAPHY

Christakis DA, Feudtner C. Ethics in a short white coat: the ethical dilemmas that medical students confront. Acad Med. 1993;68:249-54; and Feudtner C, Christakis DA. Making the rounds: the ethical development of medical students in the context of clinical rotations. Hastings Center Rep. 1994;24:6-12.

These articles examine clinical ethics dilemmas that medical students face and call for education efforts specific to students in addition to those for residents and attendings.

Rosenbaum JR, Bradley EH, Holmboe ES, et al. Sources of ethical conflict in medical housestaff training: a qualitative study. Am J Med. 2004;116:402-7.

This study examines ethical dilemmas experienced by medical house officers and found five areas of conflict: concern over telling the truth, respecting patient wishes, preventing harm, managing the limits of one's competence, and addressing the performance of someone else that is perceived to be inappropriate. Conflicts occurred between residents and attending physicians, patients or families, and other residents, and were often exacerbated by the hierarchical nature of residency training. Provides a framework to help enhance education in medical ethics and professionalism.

25

Medical Residents, Attendings, and Mistakes

Commentary by Anne-Marie J. Audet, MD, and Janet Weiner, MPH
Case History by Anne-Marie J. Audet, MD

Case History

It is late Friday night at Mercy Hospital. Martha Ellsworth, the intern on call for the general medicine service, is paged to the emergency room. There she sees Mr. Friend, age 68, who needs to be admitted for treatment of acute bronchospasm.

Mr. Friend has a history of hypertension, adult-onset diabetes mellitus, and asthma. This past week, he has been visiting his daughter, who has a dog, and he has gradually noticed increasing difficulty breathing. Tonight, he could not sleep and became progressively distressed because he could not "get any air in." He denies fever or chills but mentions having a dry cough for the past 3 days. Otherwise, he has no complaints. His medications include chlorpropamide (an oral hypoglycemic) and hydrochlorothiazide.

Dr. Ellsworth completes the history and the physical examination and draws some blood for laboratory tests. It is by now nearly 2 a.m. when she leaves Mr. Friend and writes the admission orders. She quickly checks the hospital formulary for dosage but mistakenly writes for the patient to receive chlorpromazine (a major tranquilizer) instead of chlorpropamide.

Over the weekend, Mr. Friend's respiratory status improves markedly. Late Sunday evening, as Dr. Ellsworth is preparing to present the weekend admissions at the Monday chief-of-service rounds, she reviews Mr. Friend's medication list and notices her prescription error. She immediately goes to check on the patient, who is alert and well

continued on page 155

Case History *continued from page 154*

without complaints. Dr. Ellsworth asks the nurse to do a finger stick to assess the blood glucose level and to draw blood for a stat glucose test. The finger stick indicates a glucose level of 137. The stat glucose level is 150.

Dr. Ellsworth is relieved. Fortunately, her error has not harmed Mr. Friend. But now she must deal with a more difficult problem: Whether to disclose her error to Dr. Rhys, the chief of service. Should she disclose the confusion over the name of the medication to the patient? Is she ethically responsible to disclose her error, even though no harm resulted from it?

Commentary

When should physicians disclose errors to patients and colleagues? This case study considers the issue in the context of training because how physicians handle errors made during training has clear implications for how they will handle mistakes made during the course of their careers.

Errors are inherent to the practice of medicine. They arise from medical uncertainty about diagnosis and about the risks and benefits of treatments. The environment in which decisions are made is also conducive to mistakes. Decisions often need to be made quickly, with limited knowledge, and many decisions affecting different patients need to be made under time pressures. Additionally, medical care, especially in the hospital setting, now involves many steps and people, all of whom must be well-coordinated and integrated in order to deliver high-quality care. As the system of care becomes more complex, the probability of errors increases.

Studies have looked at the frequency and the severity of errors, especially in the training setting (1,2). In one study, nearly all interns reported having made a mistake that had serious consequences for patients. While the coping and socialization processes that surround medical mistakes have been the subject of several studies (2-7), relatively little information exists on the criteria clinicians apply when they decide whether to disclose errors to their patients, colleagues, or supervising physicians. Evidence suggests that in more than half the cases residents do not discuss their mistakes with their attendings (1).

The typical mechanisms that physicians use as they face their mistakes have been well-described (2).

- Initially physicians use denial (the process by which errors are justified) because medicine is an "art" as much as a science, and because there are often no right or wrong answers, only differences of opinion.

- Then they use discounting (the process by which the responsibility for errors is assigned to external agents), blaming the system, blaming superiors for having faltered despite their greater degree of experience, blaming the disease process, blaming the inadequacies of scientific knowledge, and, finally, blaming the patient.

- Physicians may also use distancing: Because everyone makes mistakes, the personal responsibility for them is lessened. Mistakes can then be accepted as natural and understandable, and guilt can be assuaged: "I did everything I could. We all make errors. You can't know it all" (2).

Unfortunately, most of these coping mechanisms do not foster the principles of learning or those of continuous improvement that ultimately lead to better patient care. One study clearly demonstrated that such responses to mistakes (responses that often are fostered by the graduate medical education socialization process) isolate the trainees (2). These physicians come to believe that as they are singularly responsible for their actions, they should also be their own and "worst" judge. This leads them to discount attempts by others to insert them into a system of accountability. Thus most trainees, out of principles of self-reliance, choose not to disclose errors to their professional colleagues or to administrative superiors.

In our case, Dr. Ellsworth has discovered her prescription error and corrected it in a timely fashion. The patient suffered no harm from the mistake. Does Dr. Ellsworth have further responsibilities in this situation? Does she have an ethical obligation to report this to Mr. Friend, or to Dr. Rhys, the attending physician of record?

Most codes of ethics are silent when it comes to physicians' obligations to report errors to patients. The Canadian Medical Association's and the American Medical Association's codes of ethics do not directly address the duty to disclose errors to patients (8). The American College of Physicians (ACP) Ethics Manual, on the other hand, gives general guidance: "Physicians should disclose to patients information about procedural or judgment errors made in the course of care, if such information significantly affects the care of the patient. Errors do not necessarily constitute improper, negligent, or unethical behavior" (9).

Available data suggest that in most cases, physicians are reluctant to tell patients about mistakes. In one study of internal medicine house officers, only 24% told the patient or the family about mistakes affecting them (1). In a 1984 study, 78 out of 83 trainees interviewed did not believe that revealing errors to patients or to families was even an option they would consider (2).

The ACP Ethics Manual is clear about the responsibilities of physicians in training to "acknowledge their limitations and ask for help or supervision from their attending physicians, chiefs of service, or consultants when concerns arise about patient care . . . Residents must keep the attending physicians informed about each patient's hospital course and treatment plan" (9).

As she decides what to do, Dr. Ellsworth considers the consequences of disclosure and begins to weigh the benefits and the harms to herself, personally and professionally, and to her patient. She is very tempted not to tell Mr. Friend because she believes that this could result in more harm than good at this point. It would make no difference to his well-being because she made sure he was not harmed in any way by the error. She reasons that he could be distressed to learn that an error occurred and that he might lose confidence in the quality of the care provided by her and by the hospital. Indeed, trivial errors will happen in the hospital setting and do not necessarily reflect negligence.

But not disclosing the error also carries the risk of harm to the patient. Mr. Friend could discover the error on his own or learn of it from a nurse. He then would have cause to doubt the honesty and integrity of the professionals involved in his care, and the trust essential to the physician-patient relationship might be jeopardized. Without this trust, communication between physician and patient falters, and a harmful, adversarial relationship often ensues. Open communication is the best way to address the fear of litigation, given that the breakdown or the absence of an ongoing relationship between patient and physician increases the risk of legal suits.

Given these risks, in general, all relevant information should be disclosed to allow patients to participate fully in decisions about their care. This includes disclosing errors that significantly affect care. Although there is somewhat more discretion involved in disclosing trivial errors, such as a one-time substitution of a low-fat diet for a normal one, or an extra urine sample collected because of a laboratory accident, in most cases an honest discussion with the patient can and should ensue.

As a rule, physicians should begin with the premise that all errors be revealed, unless good reasons exist to do otherwise. These reasons should relate to the circumstances and the preferences of the individual patient, as gauged by the physician in the context of an established physician-patient relationship. For example, it might be appropriate to withhold knowledge of a trivial error from a patient who prefers not to hear most clinical details and only wants the big picture; it might also be acceptable in the case of a patient in an extremely fragile physical or emotional state. However, because truth-telling is so fundamental to the patient-physician relationship, the burden of proof for non-disclosure should remain great, with well-defined reasons based on the physician's best clinical judgment.

Dr. Ellsworth is reluctant to tell Dr. Rhys of her error because she is afraid that it will affect her reputation among her colleagues and might even initiate embarrassing reviews of her performance. This may compromise her competitiveness when she applies for a fellowship next year. Because the error did not hurt the patient, she figures that she would do no harm by not telling. She reasons that as long as she remains self-critical and learns from this to be very careful in the future when prescribing medications, she may have fulfilled her responsibility.

On the other hand, she feels uncomfortable with keeping this secret. By failing to reveal a mistake, even one without any consequence for patient outcome, isn't she hiding important information about the management course from the physician who is ultimately responsible for Mr. Friend's care?

Isn't she also contributing to an environment in which mistakes are kept secret, and neglecting the opportunity for everyone to learn from mistakes and to improve the quality of care? Although Dr. Ellsworth made the prescription error, others within the delivery loop failed to identify the error and prevent it. The attending did not thoroughly review the orders or the medication sheets, and the nursing staff failed to notice that the medications ordered differed from the ones that the patient was taking at the time of admission. Nor did the pharmacists notice or question the change in medication. This error could thus provide an opportunity to apply the principles of quality improvement by adopting a system-based approach to problem solving.

Dr. Ellsworth also acknowledges that her error may have important implications for the patient's future management. In the face of an acute stressor, Mr. Friend did well without his hypoglycemic medication, and may not need this drug at all. But no one will know this unless Dr. Ellsworth tells Dr. Rhys about her mistake. Dr. Rhys is ultimately accountable for the patient's care. He must trust that house staff will be completely honest about all aspects of the patient's course, as he will need this knowledge to make informed and clinically responsible management decisions.

Clinical training (clerkship, internship, residency,and fellowship) is a time when newly acquired diagnostic and therapeutic skills are put into practice. The theory of medicine, acquired in the preceding non-clinical years, is finally applied to the real world of patient care, and the uncertainties of medicine are discovered. As with any new endeavor, some mistakes will occur. They may be due to errors of judgment, lack of knowledge or technical skills, or the pressures of the practice environment.

Errors may result when communication breaks down among the numerous individuals involved in delivering care, if the system of care has inefficiencies, or just by chance. Some errors will be unavoidable or unpredictable. Whatever the cause, the severity of the error, or its consequence for the patient's outcome, the training environment should encourage learning and continuous improvement because early experiences are likely to set the tone for how physicians will deal with errors throughout their careers.

Medical practice, both during the training period and during the much longer post-training period is fraught with the possibility of making errors. The knowledge gained from them is essential to improving the quality of one's practice. This can only happen if the climate promotes free exchange of information and if errors are dealt with in a constructive, as opposed to a purely punitive, fashion. In one study of house officers' response to mistakes, only 54% discussed serious errors with their attending (1). Eighty-eight percent reported talking about an error with another colleague in a non-supervisory role, and 5% told no one about it.

The study also showed that 90% of the reported errors resulted in serious adverse outcomes: physical discomfort, emotional distress, additional therapy, additional procedures, or prolonged hospital stay. In 31% of the reported cases, the patient died. In the same study, house officers were also more likely to report constructive changes in their practice of medicine if they accepted responsibility for the mistake and discussed it with their attending.

We believe that Dr. Ellsworth should disclose her error, no matter how trivial, to her attending physician. They could then discuss the case, assess how the error affected management and outcome, and decide whether to disclose it to the patient. Mistakes that significantly affect care should always be disclosed to the patient.

As a profession, we must bring the issue of medical errors out in the open. We need to foster an environment in which physicians and patients acknowledge that errors happen and recognize that we all can and should learn from them. Just as the physician-in-training has a responsibility to discuss any mistakes with the attending of record, the attending also has the responsibility to encourage such discussions and to create a valuable learning experience.

We should strive to create an atmosphere in which errors can be resolved in an ethical and responsible manner. Truth-telling is essential to improving medical practice and to professional relationships between physicians. It forms the cornerstone of trust between physicians and patients. As a general rule, lying (even by omission) undermines these relationships and the public's trust in the medical profession. Disclosing an error to a colleague or to a patient may cause short-term discomfort, tension, or even ridicule; nevertheless, its long-term benefits, for the physician who erred, for the patient, and for the environment in which other health professionals deliver care, far outweigh the risks of secrecy.

A similar version of this case study was originally published in ACP Observer in September 1993.

REFERENCES

1. Wu AW, Folkman S, McPhee S, Lo B. Do house officers learn from their mistakes? JAMA. 1991;265:2089-94.
2. Mizrahi T. Managing medical mistakes: ideology, insularity and accountability among internists-in-training. Soc Sci Med. 1984;19:135-46.
3. Novack DH, Detering BJ, Arnold R, et al. Physicians' attitudes toward using deception to resolve difficult ethical problems. JAMA. 1989;261:2980-5.
4. Hilfiker D. Sounding board: facing our mistakes. N Engl J Med. 1984;310:118-22.
5. Christensen JF, Levinson W, Dunn P. The heart of darkness: the impact of perceived mistakes on physicians. J Gen Intern Med. 1992;7:424-31.
6. Light D. Uncertainty and control in professional training. J Health Soc Behavior. 1979;20:310-22.
7. Bosk CL. Forgive and Remember: Managing Medical Failure. Chicago: University of Chicago Press; 1979.
8. Warner E. Telling patients about medical negligence. Can Med Assoc J. 1983; 129:366-8.
9. American College of Physicians. Ethics Manual, 3rd ed. Ann Intern Med. 1992;117: 947-60.

ANNOTATED BIBLIOGRAPHY

Crook ED, Stellini M, Levine D, et al. Medical errors and the trainee: ethical concerns. Am J Med Sci. 2004;327:33-7.

In teaching hospitals, medical students and house officers often observe or make mistakes. Although disclosure is the ethical standard, the consequences of disclosure are often feared. This article stresses that future physicians must have appropriate training, mentoring, and support when dealing with errors.

Wu AW, Folkman S, McPhee S, Lo B. Do house officers learn from their mistakes? JAMA. 1991;265:2089-94.

The internal medicine house officers who acknowledged, accepted responsibility for, and discussed their mistakes were more likely to make constructive changes in their practice.

Part IV

THE BUSINESS OF MEDICINE: EFFECTS ON THE PATIENT-PHYSICIAN RELATIONSHIP

The practice of medicine does not take place in a vacuum. Its occurs within a context—the health care system—and within our uniquely American culture.

Economic issues have implications for the delivery of care. Three are dealt with in Part IV. First, generalist-specialist relations are examined in the context of health plan incentives. Next, financial incentives and their potential influence on clinical decision-making in both managed care and fee-for-service indemnity settings are considered. The final chapter looks at issues raised by the role the drug industry has played in the financial support of continuing medical education activities and its potential effects on patient care.

26

Are Health Plan Incentives Hurting Generalist-Specialist Relationships?

Commentary and Case History by Daniel P. Sulmasy, OFM, MD, PhD

Case History

Judy Judkins, an invasive cardiologist, has been in private practice for 20 years. She belongs to a busy group of five cardiologists in Pottertown, an industrial city. The city's largest manufacturer, UniCorp, which employs 20% of Pottertown's work force, recently switched health insurance plans to reduce its health care costs. It now uses CareUSA, a capitated plan.

CareUSA tries to contain costs by making its physicians financially responsible for minimizing unnecessary referrals, tests, and treatments. The HMO withholds 15% of primary care physicians' pay and returns it only if physicians meet expenditure targets for tests, treatments, and referrals. Like most physicians in the area, Dr. Judkins' group signs on with CareUSA because the plan has such a large patient base.

A 58-year-old UniCorp employee, Guy Montag, presents with chest pain and anterior ST-segment elevations at Good Samaritan Hospital. He is treated with aspirin and TPA and admitted to the coronary care unit under Dr. Judkins' care.

CareUSA certifies the admission and tells Dr. Judkins that Mr. Montag's primary care internist, Dr. Kenobe, will contact her. Dr. Kenobe visits later that day and informs Dr. Judkins that he will assume care as the attending of record, but that Dr. Judkins can consult.

Dr. Judkins is a bit annoyed, as she is accustomed to being the attending of record for patients she cares for in the coronary unit. She has not worked with Dr. Kenobe before, however, so she doesn't voice her frustrations.

continued on page 164

Case History *continued from page 163*

Mr. Montag's post-MI course is relatively uncomplicated, and he is discharged on atenolol and aspirin after a negative low-level stress test. As part of the patient's post-discharge plans, Dr. Judkins plans to retest his lipids to assess the need for cholesterol-lowering agents. She also plans to perform a symptom-limited full stress test in 2 weeks to assess Mr. Montag's preparedness for a phase II cardiac rehabilitation program.

Dr. Judkins writes an order for an appointment to perform the follow-up stress test in her office and to supervise the phase II rehabilitation program. Later that morning, however, she receives a call from Dr. Kenobe. He thanks her for her concern but says that he will perform the stress test in his office. He also explains that he will supervise the rehabilitation program and will contact Dr. Judkins if any problems arise.

Dr. Judkins begins to wonder whether the managed care environment and CareUSA's financial incentives are having an adverse impact on Mr. Montag's care, as well as on her relationships with primary care physicians in general. She wonders whether what she sees happening is ethical.

Commentary

Physicians' primary ethical responsibility is to decide on the proper care for their individual patients. However, this care does not take place in a vacuum (1). Beyond face-to-face encounters with individual patients, physicians also have moral responsibilities toward other patients, ethical duties to insurers, and responsibilities to society as a whole.

Medicine today is no longer an individual enterprise. Generalists and specialists must cooperate now more than ever to optimize patient care. Ethical and contractual obligations to HMOs add another layer of moral responsibility and may complicate relationships between specialists and generalists. Dr. Judkins' interaction with Dr. Kenobe highlights many of these issues.

Competence and Ethical Obligations

Physicians have an ethical duty not only to provide the care for which they have been trained, but also to avoid offering care that they have not been adequately trained to administer. The Hippocratic oath states that one should "forswear the use of the knife in deference to those who are skilled in its use." Many ethicists interpret this as a pledge that physicians should not exceed their competence.

If Dr. Kenobe can competently supervise exercise tolerance testing and cardiac rehabilitation, there is nothing wrong with his providing that care. An ethical problem exists only if he exceeds the boundaries of his competence to increase his income under CareUSA's capitation system.

Some ethicists worry that managed care is forcing generalists to act as marginal specialists and specialists to behave like marginal generalists (2). Some general internists complain that they are being asked to stretch the care they deliver beyond their competency (3). Dr. Judkins' moral disquiet about Dr. Kenobe's decision to provide all Mr. Montag's post-MI care reflects her concerns that he is acting as a "marginal specialist."

A controversial body of literature has suggested that patients who receive post-MI care from a cardiologist receive "more appropriate" care than those cared for by generalists (4-7). Critics, however, have argued that differences in outcomes are sometimes due to the treating physician's caseload and experience, factors that can operate independently of the physician's specialty (8). Others have suggested that the most appropriate care takes place in settings where generalists and specialists collaborate closely (9,10).

It is often said that generalists tend to underutilize treatments and procedures and specialists tend to overutilize them (5). The practices of individual specialists and generalists vary widely, however, and physicians should avoid stereotyping. What matters most is the competence of the care rendered, not the type of physician who provides the care.

The critical ethical point is that the patient's care, whether provided by a generalist or a specialist or both, should be medically appropriate. Mr. Montag received appropriate therapy and the plans for his future care were appropriate.

Generalist-Specialist Communication

While communication between generalists and specialists is an area of concern in all practice environments, the managed care setting (with the possible exception of the staff model HMO) poses unique barriers to effective communication between generalists and specialists (11).

Because health plans' physician panels change frequently, generalists often find it difficult to maintain close working relationships with specialists (12). Drs. Judkins and Kenobe, for instance, have never worked together before and don't know each other's style of practice.

As generalists are forced to refer patients to specialists they do not know, they often find it difficult to call for advice that might forestall a referral. Generalists also find it difficult to interpret advice from specialists who are strangers to them.

Collaboration between generalists and specialists improves when physicians understand each other's style. ("That Judy Judkins is conservative. She caths only when it's absolutely necessary.") Dr. Judkins, for instance, might be less worried if she knew that Dr. Kenobe is highly skilled at supervising exercise tolerance testing and that he would seek appropriate assistance if anything were to go awry.

One solution might be to institute a policy that encourages physicians to talk to each other by telephone each time a consultation is requested. Such a policy would facilitate personal contact.

Patient-Physician Communication

Physicians have a duty to communicate not only with other physicians but also with patients (1). Because respect for patient autonomy demands that patients be involved in decision-making, Dr. Kenobe should discuss options with Mr. Montag.

Another major issue is whether Dr. Kenobe should disclose CareUSA's financial incentives designed to discourage him from referring patients to specialty physicians. While some managed care plans may explicitly or subtly disapprove of such disclosures, many physicians believe they have an ethical duty to disclose financial incentives (13).

Generalists may want to use "curbside consults" to informally bring specialists into the patient's care, but such consults should be avoided. Because taking a history requires direct interaction, there may be cases in which specialists can render proper advice only by talking directly to the patient.

Perhaps all cases do not require patients to see a specialist in person. A phone call from the specialist to the patient might suffice in some instances. In this case, for instance, Dr. Judkins might simply ask Dr. Kenobe for an opportunity to speak to Mr. Montag directly over the phone.

Cost-Containment

Both Drs. Judkins and Kenobe have a duty to patients and to society to avoid unnecessary and expensive tests and treatments. They might, for instance, consider whether exercise testing is necessary before proceeding with cardiac rehabilitation (14).

Physicians have a duty to be good stewards of society's health care resources, but they also must be sure that cost-containment measures do not adversely affect patient care (1). While Mr. Montag does not appear to have been adversely affected by Dr. Kenobe's decision not to refer to a cardiologist, there were evident tensions between Dr. Kenobe and Dr. Judkins that could lead to adverse effects in the future.

Both physicians should make special efforts to communicate with each other effectively in the future. They should also commit to working toward health care reform that not only controls health care costs but also facilitates generalist-specialist communication and optimizes patient care.

A similar version of this case study was originally published in ACP Observer in June 2001.

REFERENCES

1. American College of Physicians. Ethics Manual, 4th ed. Ann Intern Med. 1998; 128:576-94.
2. Pellegrino ED. Managed care at the bedside: how do we look in the moral mirror? Kennedy Institute of Ethics Journal. 1997;7:321-30.
3. St Peter RF, Reed MC, Kemper P, Blumenthal D. Changes in the scope of care provided by primary care physicians. N Engl J Med. 1999;341:1980-5.
4. Ayanian JZ, Hauptman P, Guadagnoli E, et al. Knowledge and practices of generalist and specialist physicians regarding drug therapy for acute myocardial infarction. N Engl J Med. 1994;331:1136-42.
5. Donohoe MT. Comparing generalist and specialty care: discrepancies, deficiencies, and excesses. Arch Intern Med. 1998;158:1596-1608.
6. Ayanian JZ, Guadagnoli E, McNeil BJ, Cleary PD. Treatment and outcomes of acute myocardial infarction among patients of cardiologists and generalist physicians. Arch Intern Med. 1997;157:2570-6.
7. Casale PN, Jones JL, Wolf FE, et al. Patients treated by cardiologists have lower in-hospital mortality for acute myocardial infarction. J Am Coll Cardiol. 1998;32:885-9.
8. Nash IS, Corrato RR, Dlutowski MJ, Nash DB. Generalist versus specialist care for acute myocardial infarction. Am J Cardiol. 1999;83:650-4.
9. Wilson DJ, Soumerai SB, McLaughlin TJ, et al. Consultation between cardiologists and generalists in the management of acute myocardial infarction: implications for quality of care. Arch Intern Med. 1998;158:1778-83.
10. Ayanian JZ. Generalists and specialists caring for patients with heart disease: united we stand, divided we fall. Am J Med. 2000;108:259-61.
11. Roulidis ZC, Schulman KA. Physician communication in managed care organizations: opinions of primary care physicians. J Fam Pract. 1994;39:446-51.
12. Flock SA, Stange KC, Zyzanski SJ. The impact of insurance type and forced discontinuity on the delivery of primary care. J Fam Pract. 1997;45:129-35.
13. Sulmasy DP, Bloch MG, Mitchell JM, Hadley J. Physicians' ethical beliefs about cost-control arrangements. Arch Intern Med. 2000;160:649-57.
14. McConnell TR, Klinger TA, Gardner JK, et al. Cardiac rehabilitation without exercise tests for post-myocardial infarction and post-bypass surgery patients. J Cardiopulm Rehab. 1998;18:458-63.

ANNOTATED BIBLIOGRAPHY

Bodenheimer T, Lo B, Casalino L. Primary care physicians should be coordinators, not gatekeepers. JAMA. 1999;281:2045-9.

This paper advises that in order to improve quality of care, primary care physicians should serve as coordinators of primary and specialty care in a managed care system. Describes proposals to redesign primary care network, referral and payment processes.

Povar GJ, Blumen H, Daniel J, et al. Ethics in practice: managed care and the changing health care environment. Medicine as a Profession Managed Care Ethics Working Group Statement. Ann Intern Med. 2004;141:131-5.

Explores the impact of a changing health care environment on patient-physician relationships and how to best apply the principles of professionalism in that environment. This statement, developed by patients, patient advocates, clinicians, health plan leadership, and medical ethicists, offers guidance on preserving the patient-clinician relationship, patient rights and responsibilities, confidentiality and privacy, resource allocation and stewardship, and the obligation of health plans to foster an ethical environment for the delivery of care, among other issues.

27

Financial Incentives and Physician Decision-Making

Commentary by Lois Snyder, JD
Case History by Alan L. Hillman, MD, MBA

Case History

Ted and Ned are 46-year-old, asymptomatic, sedentary identical twins. Both are executives in local corporations. Former smokers (both smoked about one-half pack per day from their late teens to their early 30s, when they quit as a New Year's resolution), they have been generally healthy except for mild obesity, secondary to many executive lunches. As a New Year's resolution for 1990, Ted and Ned agree to join a local gym to "tone up" and get back in shape. Both had been college athletes. The gym required a note from each man's doctor before they could start the exercise program, but no specific tests were mandated.

Ted had enrolled in GreatCare, an IPA-model HMO, because he liked the "comprehensive care" concept, including an emphasis on prevention and wellness. He also valued the idea of no out-of-pocket health care costs other than the premium deducted from his paycheck. Because it is an IPA-model HMO, in which the HMO contracts with independent providers in private practice, Ted was able to select a local physician about whom he had heard good things.

Unbeknownst to Ted, his physician had agreed to certain contractual arrangements with the HMO. Among them were a 15% discount on his usual fees and an additional 15% withholding. The HMO would return the 15% withholding to the physician only if his referral account for specialist services and laboratory tests had a surplus at the end of the year. If the referral account had a surplus, the physician would get

continued on page 170

Case History *continued from page 169*

his withheld funds and a bonus equal to half of his share of any surplus in the referral pool. The HMO, which had grouped Ted's physician with four others in his community as a risk pool, provided him with the names, addresses and telephone numbers of these other physicians and encouraged him to contact the group to "discuss the use of referral funds from their aggregate pool."

Ned had elected traditional indemnity fee-for-service health care insurance, in which his premiums and out-of-pocket payments were higher than Ted's. He felt that it was important to retain complete freedom of choice with respect to doctors, despite the somewhat higher overall costs. As is usual in traditional fee-for-service health care, Ned's doctor is paid for each patient visit and every service performed.

Ted and Ned met at the gym for their first joint workout. Ned mentioned that his physician would not write a note for him to start the program without first performing an ECG and exercise tolerance test (results of which were normal). Ned takes some pride in what he considers to be his doctor's comprehensive approach to his health care, and the extra attention he got for clearance for the exercise program. Ted wants to know why his doctor hadn't ordered the tests. After some thought, Ned begins to wonder if the expensive and time-consuming tests he received really were needed. Both brothers are confused.

Commentary

The physician's primary obligations are to the patient, not to the system under which he provides care, and certainly not to the physician's own pocketbook. It is obviously easiest to follow the ethical course under medically clear circumstances: An exercise tolerance test would be medically unnecessary for a 20-year-old college athlete, about to join a gym, who has no risk factors.

Most situations require physician judgment as to whether an intervention or test is appropriate given the individual patient. The objectivity of physician discretion must not be allowed to be affected by external forces.

The American College of Physicians Ethics Manual states: "The welfare of the patient must at all times be paramount, and the physician must insist that the medically appropriate level of care takes primacy over fiscal considerations . . . The guiding principle should always be care consistent with humanistic, scientific and efficient medicine . . . In the final analysis, no external factors should interfere with the dedication of the physician to provide optimal care for his or her patient" (1).

In addition to obvious influences on behavior, physicians must be aware of more subtle influences that could affect judgment when the best clinical decision for an individual patient is unclear; for example, in the fee-for-service setting a physician may too quickly recommend a test or procedure, while the HMO physician may adopt a wait-and-see approach for too long (2).

The patient-physician relationship necessarily involves unequal partners. Vulnerable patients entrust their health and lives to physicians, the keepers and communicators of medical knowledge. Patients have the right to make informed decisions about their care. But physicians have the power to influence decision-making.

With fee-for-service, more tests mean more fees. Physicians must be aware of, and seek to avoid, the "more is better" philosophy that this setting might implicitly encourage. Some commentators have said that potential conflict is easier for the patient to see in this setting; patients know that the more the doctor does, the more he gets paid. The patient's ability to verify the medical need for a service by getting a second opinion can serve as a check on physician behavior (3).

That certainly holds true regarding the need for a major operation, but Ned has no reason to question his doctor's judgment that exercise testing is required in order to evaluate whether he can join the gym. And even if the second opinion "check" theory were applicable more often, it would not convert behavior that was ethically unacceptable into ethically acceptable behavior.

In the HMO setting, if a medically needed service is denied because incentives distort physician judgment, rather than merely encourage cost-effective care, the patient may be unlikely to know it. Here, there has been no discourse between physician and patient. In the fee-for-service context something affirmative has to happen before the physician profits: the physician must propose the service and perform the test. If the physician refers the patient elsewhere, and if something other than appropriate care motivates the referral, it raises issues ranging from fee-splitting to unnecessary referrals.

In the HMO setting, the patient may not know a type of care is being omitted. Some patients may question what they see as a lack of care, if they expected to undergo a test or receive a prescription, for example, but others may not know what care is missing.

A number of lawsuits naming HMOs as defendants are now making their way through the courts. Plaintiffs have alleged that HMO incentive systems, which had not been disclosed to them, compromised the independent judgment of primary physicians, resulting in poor health care services. Physicians can themselves end up as defendants. In the fee-for-service setting, fear of lawsuits has been cited as the basis for so-called "defensive medicine," but this does not justify providing unnecessary care. The practice and documentation of medically appropriate care remain the best defense in a medical malpractice action. The threat of lawsuits should no more affect care than clinical judgment should be distorted by financial incentives.

In a fee-for-service practice, a physician may consciously or unconsciously over-test. In using tests appropriately, physicians must look not only at the immediate costs of a test, but consider that additional expenses can mount in the follow-up of a result that turns out to be a false-positive. Also important are the potential medical complications in the performance of the original test or follow-up, and the anxiety patients may suffer while waiting to find out if they actually have the disease or condition. These are reasons that ACP and others have been developing guidelines for the use of common tests in screening, case-finding, diagnosis, and management of disease.

However, a physician attempting to care for Ted or Ned in accordance with ACP medical necessity guidelines (Screening for Asymptomatic Coronary Artery Disease: Exercise Stress Testing; and Screening for Asymptomatic CAD: The Resting Electrocardiogram [4]) would be in a gray zone and would have to rely on his or her individual judgment.

The exercise stress testing guidelines state: "Exercise testing is not recommended as a routine screening procedure in adults with no evidence of coronary heart disease and no risk factors . . . Some asymptomatic persons may have particular reasons to consider exercise stress testing for coronary artery disease. Some persons are especially likely to have the disease because of increased age, male gender, and at least one other risk factor (family history of CAD, cigarette smoking, diabetes mellitus, systolic blood pressure greater than 140 mm Hg, hypercholesterolemia, or a cholesterol to HDL ratio of more than 6.0). Other persons who should be tested are those who have an occupation that puts others at risk (for example, bus drivers or airline pilots) or are sedentary and about to begin a program of physical conditioning. There is insufficient evidence to make a strong recommendation for or against use of routine stress testing in these groups" (4).

Similarly, the resting electrocardiogram guidelines list the above risk factors for CAD and state: "The resting ECG is not recommended as a routine practice in people who are under age 65 and do not have evidence for cardiovascular disease or its risk factors. However, it may be appropriate in selected patients, especially in situations where the published evidence is not decisive" (4).

The fact that the brothers are former cigarette smokers could put them at increased risk for coronary artery disease, but this is not as clear-cut as it would be for current smokers, or those who smoked several packs per day or quit more recently. The sedentary nature and mild obesity of each patient, in addition to the nature of the exercise program each is about to start, are additional considerations for the physicians to evaluate. Decision-making is also affected by variation in the information elicited by different physicians in the history and physical examination. Styles of diagnosis and management, personalities, and patient needs and preferences all can affect medical choices.

As long as these and other medical factors were the reasons for the decisions regarding testing, the best interest of each patient is motivating each physician. As it turns out, each doctor's income was enhanced here because the fee-for-service physician performed the tests on Ned, while the HMO doctor, whose take-home pay could be reduced had he ordered the tests, did not order them for Ted.

Finally, the comparison of the care they received has left both Ned and Ted somewhat confused. Patients need to be able to have confidence in the care they receive and must always be fully informed about the medical care that they accept. Given the circumstances, Ted's physician probably need not have explained why he was not doing tests he felt were not medically indicated (unless the patient had asked about it specifically), although he should explain his reasoning fully when and if Ted raises this at his next visit. Likewise, Ned's physician may need to go into greater detail at Ned's request. Decisions that patients perceive as conflicts of interest on the part of their physicians can undermine the patient-physician relationship.

Conclusion

Physicians have an ethical duty to be aware of the financial incentives of the system in which they practice and the possibility of obvious and subtle influences. Disclosing financial incentives and interests might provide patients with needed information, although this is not necessarily a remedy to conflicts. Little has been written about the mechanics of disclosure such as how and what information should be presented and oversight measures to ensure compliance (5).

Disclosure might range from physician statements about ownership interests in a laboratory or other health care entity to which the physician refers patients, to explanations of the incentives of particular practice settings. Physicians are not relieved of their obligation to serve the best interests of their patients, however, whether or not they, or the organizations for which they work, disclose the relevant financial incentives under which they practice medicine.

A similar version of this case study was originally published in ACP Observer in October 1990.

References

1. American College of Physicians. Ethics Manual, 2nd ed, Part 1: History; The Patient; Other Physicians. Ann Intern Med. 1989;111:245-52; Part 2: The Physician and Society; Research: Life-Sustaining Treatment; Other Issues. Ann Intern Med. 1989;111:327-35.
2. Hillman A. Health maintenance organizations, financial incentives and physicians' judgments. Ann Intern Med. 1990;112:891-3.
3. Morreim H. Conflicts of interest: profits and problems in physician referrals. JAMA. 1989;262:390-4.
4. Eddy DM. Common Screening Tests. Philadelphia: American College of Physicians; 1991.
5. Rodwin M. Physicians' conflicts of interest: the limitations of disclosure. N Engl J Med. 1989;321:1405-8.

Annotated Bibliography

Keating NL, Landon BE, Ayanian JZ, et al. Practice, clinical management, and financial arrangements of practicing generalists. J Gen Intern Med. 2004;19:410-8.

Pressures to limit referrals and to see more patients are common, particularly among physicians paid based on productivity or capitation. These pressures are associated with career dissatisfaction and professionalism concerns.

Povar GJ, Blumen H, Daniel J, et al. Ethics in practice: managed care and the changing health care environment. Medicine as a Profession Managed Care Ethics Working Group Statement. Ann Intern Med. 2004;141:131-5.

Explores the impact of a changing health care environment on patient-physician relationships and how to best apply the principles of professionalism in that environment. This statement, developed by patients, patient advocates, clinicians, health plan leadership, and medical ethicists, offers guidance on preserving the patient-clinician relationship, patient rights and responsibilities, confidentiality and privacy, resource allocation and stewardship, and the obligation of health plans to foster an ethical environment for the delivery of care, among other issues.

Rodwin MA. Conflicts in managed care. N Engl J Med. 1995;332:606-6.

Describes a "conflict" model of managed care, its ethical and legal implications, and methods for dealing with the conflicts.

Rodwin MA. Financial incentives for doctors. BMJ. 2004;328:1328-9.

This article argues that financial incentives for doctors have their place when used for appropriate goals, such as promoting high-quality patient-centered care and the efficient use of resources. The challenge is to minimize or avoid the perverse effects of incentives and their problems and risks. Incentives should be viewed like drugs: a powerful tool that can be beneficial but also dangerous. Concludes that society should control the use of incentives for doctors.

Thompson DF. Understanding financial conflicts of interest. N Engl J Med. 1993;329: 573-6.

Defines conflict of interest broadly and reviews potential standards for assessing conflicts and remedies, including individual provider discretion, professional and governmental regulation, and disclosure. Calls for clear guidelines for avoiding conflicts.

28

Pharmaceutical Industry Support of Continuing Medical Education

Commentaries by Janet Weiner, MPH, Lois Snyder, JD,
Kathleen L. Egan, PhD, and Frank F. Davidoff, MD
Case History by Janet Weiner, MPH, and Lois Snyder, JD

Case History

Dr. Sira Assad is a general internist practicing in a working class neighborhood of a small city. At the end of a busy day, she emerges from the exam room in great frustration after seeing a long-time patient, Ms. Bertha Lake. Ms. Lake, a 67-year-old woman with hypertension, follows her slowly to her office.

"Ms. Lake, you need to be taking this medication every day. Not every other day, not half the dosage. Your blood pressure is 185/100, even higher than it was last month."

Ms. Lake shares her ongoing concerns and anxiety about her finances. "But Dr. Assad, I can't afford that stuff. I live on a fixed income and the pills cost $70 a month. Medicare doesn't cover them. Can't we go with something cheaper?"

Dr. Assad remembers that she tried other, less expensive drugs, but they did not result in adequate control of Ms. Lake's blood pressure. Dr. Assad feels helpless. "Here are some free samples. They'll tide you over until you can find a way to pay for the drug. It's very important to get back on it and stay on it." Dr. Assad gives Ms. Lake the rest of the samples left by the drug company representative (a 3-week supply) and worries about what will happen when they run out. She gives her patient a new prescription and a return appointment and tells her to call if she can't fill the prescription.

After Ms. Lake leaves, Dr. Assad calls the drug representative to

continued on page 177

Case History *continued from page 176*

ask for more samples. The drug rep says that he can't replenish her supply because he did so just 2 days before. Dr. Assad asks whether the company has a program for supplying indigent patients with drugs at no or reduced cost. The rep replies that the company does not have a program in place but is in the process of devising one.

The next morning, after visiting her patients at the hospital, Dr. Assad gets a call from the hospital's director of medical education (DME), Dr. Gabriel Fowler. Like Dr. Assad, Dr. Fowler is a busy private practitioner. Serving as chair of the medical education committee is part of his "payback" to the hospital. Dr. Fowler is taking his responsibilities as DME quite seriously and has spent many hours in the last few months planning a continuing medical education (CME) program to update primary care physicians on cardiovascular disease. He has procured an educational grant from a drug company for the program and has insisted upon maintaining control of the program content and the speakers invited. His mission today is to spread the word to his colleagues and to urge them to register for the program.

Dr. Assad listens as Dr. Fowler reminds her about the deadline to register for this full-day program, to be held at a convenient local hotel. Dr. Assad, after hearing the topics and the faculty, signs up. The program has no registration fee and includes a full dinner.

A few weeks later, Dr. Assad is listening to an excellent lecture in the CME program when her beeper goes off. Ms. Lake has called, scared and wanting to know if she should go to the hospital. Suddenly she has found that she can't speak clearly and her right hand is clumsy. Her face feels funny and looks "off balance" in the mirror. Thoughts race through Dr. Assad's mind: Is this an accomplished stroke or a transient ischemic attack? Is this happening because Ms. Lake has just run out of medication? Or is Ms. Lake paying the price for the inadequate control of her blood pressure over time?

On the way to meet her patient at the emergency room, Dr. Assad looks at the program materials in her hands and realizes that the pharmaceutical company supporter of the CME program produces the drug that Ms. Lake can't afford. She suddenly feels confused and resentful. How much cheaper would the drug be if the company didn't spend so much on glossy advertisements, brochures, handouts, pens, samples, and fancy CME dinners? Why are these drug reps milling around the reception area at the CME conference? Why is her hospital

continued on page 178

Case History *continued from page 177*

accepting this kind of largess? Is she being taken advantage of? Is her patient paying, indirectly, for the amenities of this meeting?

At the hospital the next day, Dr. Assad runs into Dr. Fowler and voices her discomfort with the circumstances of the meeting. She is surprised when Dr. Fowler becomes impatient.

"How do you expect a small hospital to pay for such a high-quality meeting?" he asked. "You know how expensive it is to print and mail brochures, to bring in faculty from leading academic medical centers, to rent the space and provide decent meals. The companies want to pay for it, and good CME is hard to find near home. You should be glad we can arrange it!"

Dr. Assad is not convinced. When it is her turn to direct medical education at the hospital, she wonders, will she do things differently?

Commentary on Dr. Assad's Situation

In her proper role as an advocate for her patient, Dr. Assad is questioning the actions of both the pharmaceutical industry and the medical profession within a system that fails to guarantee that medically necessary drugs will be affordable for all people. She is making connections between seemingly unconnected events in her professional life that may be contributing to a medically and ethically unacceptable outcome for her patient.

It is morally unacceptable for money to stand in the way of Ms. Lake's ability to obtain a needed drug. And yet this is a reality for her and many other patients. Some would argue that this is a result of gaps in insurance coverage, while others argue that the high price of drugs is primarily to blame. Our health care system is flawed on both counts; it is likely that high prices contribute to the widening gaps in insurance, and both factors combine to create the economic and moral dilemma we face.

In 1988, retail spending for prescription drugs amounted to $27.1 billion, 56% of which was paid for by consumers out-of-pocket (1). The elderly, who constituted 12% of the total population in 1988, accounted for 35% of prescription drug expenditures (1). Meanwhile, 16 pharmaceutical companies surveyed by the Senate spent $85.9 million in 1988 sponsoring 34,688 scientific symposia (2). In the same year, the pharmaceutical industry was estimated to spend about $200 million a year on medical education (as distinct from promotional activities) (3).

In general, the industry is estimated to spend more than $10 billion a year on promotion, which exceeds spending on research by $1 billion (4). Overall, the drug industry spends about 24% of its sales revenue on promotion (2).

Promotion or Education?

The ethics of industry-supported CME have mostly focused on the distinction between promotion and education, emphasizing the need to resist promotional bias and maintain the scientific integrity of the programs. The importance of the CME provider controlling the content of educational programs has been underscored most recently by the FDA (5), but also by the American Medical Association (6), the American College of Physicians (3), and many others. However, existing ethical guidelines are noticeably silent on the question of the physician's role in influencing the affordability of prescription drugs. Beyond being cost-conscious and prescribing only medically necessary drugs, does the physician have any obligation to influence the broader forces that result in drug prices beyond the means of many patients?

Dr. Assad is aware that many drug companies offer indigent patient programs. In a 1992 directory published by the Pharmaceutical Manufacturers Association, 59 companies listed indigent programs covering a varying number of drugs and having different eligibility requirements (7). Dr. Assad has used this service in the past, and a few of her desperately poor patients have benefited. But from experience she knows that these programs can have cumbersome paperwork requirements for certifying eligibility and for continuous re-certification, and often do not serve people just beyond the poverty level. She is convinced that these programs, although they respond compassionately to some people in desperate need, do not meet the needs of many people who cannot afford expensive medications.

Dr. Assad has noted that the pharmaceutical companies spend considerable funds on physicians and physician groups. The money is spent on detailing, distribution of free samples, advertising (including promotional booths and materials at educational functions), and direct support for educational activities. The companies set the prices of their drugs, and these pricing decisions have led to a relatively high level of industry profits, according to some analysts (8,9). Given these business decisions, it is not unreasonable to conclude that pharmaceutical companies pass the costs of their relationships with the medical profession on to consumers through inflated prices.

One might immediately respond that lessening support of CME does not automatically mean that drug prices will be lower. CME providers will have no control over the funds that they refuse and therefore, on a practical level, cannot ensure that drugs will become more affordable for patients. Furthermore, both patients and physicians may lose the benefits derived from this spending, such as quality CME programs and free samples for patients.

The controversy has led a number of commentators to question the need for the industry's support of CME. "The pharmaceutical industry must promote and sell its products. Medical education must educate and avoid promotion. We are in a quandary of our own making because we have decided that we cannot afford to educate ourselves without this industry's support" (10).

Another physician, Dr. Douglas Waud, writes, "I believe physicians can buy books and attend meetings without fear of landing in the poorhouse" (11). He maintains that subsidies for meetings are "bribes" that free up physicians' own money for other purposes. Because this money comes out of the pockets of patients, Dr. Waud finds it "at odds with the physician's responsibility to act in the best interests of the patient."

And what about the free samples that Dr. Assad gave to Ms. Lake? She has reason to question the benefits of this aspect of pharmaceutical promotion as well. Manufacturers distributed 2.4 billion samples in 1988, yet there is little published information on the clinical use of sample medications (2). A recent study concluded that although a majority of medications dispensed were given to patients, approximately one third of the value of the medications either went to physicians and their families or had an unknown destination (12). The authors found a high association between sample dispensing and simultaneous prescribing of the same brand-name drug, which supports the contention that sampling influences physician-prescribing habits. Although this influence might not be the decisive factor for Dr. Assad and Ms. Lake in our case, the overall effect on prescribing patterns cannot be ignored. Combine this effect with evidence that most physicians do not know the actual prices of drugs, and it is easy to see how samples may actually contribute to higher out-of-pocket drug costs for patients (13).

Are physicians prepared to forego CME subsidies, drug samples, and other amenities provided by industry? And if so, can physicians at the same time pressure the pharmaceutical companies to lower their prices? The answers to both questions are not clear. However, Dr. Assad will surely discover them if she attempts to conduct CME programs without industry support. Given the social, medical, and economic costs to patients, efforts to minimize the medical profession's reliance on industry support are worth a try.

Commentary on Dr. Fowler's Situation

Dr. Fowler is somewhat taken aback by Dr. Assad's reaction to the meeting. Is she trying to say that industry support of CME should be banned? He does not agree. For him, the issue is not whether there should be any relationship between industry and physicians but, rather, how to define that relationship for the good of patients. "A responsible and productive alliance between the medical profession and the pharmaceutical industry is unquestionably beneficial to medical progress . . . partnered activities offer important opportunities to impartially advance the state of medical practice and thus improve patient care" (3).

As director of medical education, Dr. Fowler has closely followed issues regarding the ethics of industry-supported CME and industry gifts to doctors, including the development of guidelines by the FDA, the Accreditation Council for Continuing Medical Education (14), the American Medical Association, the Pharmaceutical Manufacturers Association (15), the American College of Physicians, and others. For these groups and for Dr. Fowler, the ethical issues surrounding CME are about distinguishing between education and promotion and maintaining the scientific integrity of programs.

Medical education and scientific exchange are important endeavors that lead to improved patient care. Promotion of particular products, on the other hand, should be labeled as such and regulated; subtle or disguised promotion that introduces bias into supposedly objective publications and programs should be eliminated. Physicians have an ethical obligation to their patients, to the profession, and to society to preserve the objectivity of clinical judgment and avoid even the appearance of outside influences. They must confront issues of potential bias in evaluating medical information whatever the source, be it academic, professional, or commercial.

In the CME context, Dr. Fowler believes that physicians must be especially sensitive to the need to eliminate, or at a minimum to control, potential bias in any commercial presentation of medical information. To that end, he has scrupulously followed the guidelines of the groups noted above and maintained complete control over program content and faculty selection. When the drug company approached him with available funds, he accepted on the condition that he and his colleagues choose topics and faculty.

They settled on a comprehensive update on cardiovascular disease, a topic of many dimensions, great relevance in the community, and wide appeal to the medical staff. Speakers were required to disclose any financial or other interests that might affect their presentation. The drug company had no role in the course budget, honoraria payment, or selection of who attended the program. Company funding was disclosed. Drug reps and promotional materials were not permitted in or near the meeting room. Dr. Fowler considers the hospitality provided to be modest. He feels safe in declaring that the program was not biased by the source of funding.

Would Prices Change?

Why is Dr. Assad so concerned? Dr. Fowler wonders. Does shse believe that decreasing or ending industry support for CME will automatically mean that drug prices will be lower? The amount of money spent on CME by industry ($200 million) does not even begin to compare to what companies collectively spend on promotion in the United States: some $10 billion a year (16). And as a percentage of the $27 billion in retail spending on prescription drugs, it amounts to less than 1%.

Had he refused the funds, the company likely would have just gone to another hospital. This would put Dr. Fowler's medical staff, for whom he is charged with providing quality CME, at a disadvantage. The patients, who benefit from their doctors' continuing education, would also lose out. Could they have put on a program of this quality with their own resources? Should they?

The issue of drug prices must be seen in the larger context of universal access to health care. Are physicians obligated to influence the broader forces that result in drug prices beyond the means of patients? Dr. Fowler believes the answer is yes, to the extent that physicians must be advocates for the health of the public, especially within the current debate about health care reform. For Dr. Fowler, though, the direct care of patients is the ethical issue, and one that physicians can do something about. But many physicians do not even accept Medicare or Medicaid patients into their practices, let alone uninsured people. "What about their care?" he remembers asking during a heated discussion with a colleague. Ethics, it seems to Dr. Fowler, begin at home, in the physician's office.

On further reflection, Dr. Fowler is reminded of the reaction of many physicians when medical groups and others first started issuing guidelines for physician/pharmaceutical relations. No group had proposed that pharmaceutical support be branded as unethical per se and banned altogether. Instead, guidelines were suggested to help define and ensure ethical relations and behavior. Even so, many physicians felt that they were being treated as though they were "guilty until proven innocent." Wrote Julian Berman, of Coral Springs, Florida:

"I am not at an academic medical center. The medical education available to me without leaving the office for a week to travel . . . consists of pharmaceutical company–sponsored lectures given by experts at our local hospitals and restaurants, and weekend meetings in pleasant surroundings that feature nationally known speakers . . . I am generally sick and tired of having my ethical sense denigrated by editors and academics who do not know me, how I make my decisions, or, for that matter, what decisions I make. To answer the question posed in the American College of Physicians' position paper (Physicians and the Pharmaceutical Industry [3]), I would not mind at all if my arrangements with the pharmaceutical industry were generally known" (17).

Dr. Berman was referring to the Royal College of Physicians guideline, "Would I be willing to have this arrangement generally known?", which was adopted by the American College of Physicians, along with the additional query, "What would the public or my patients think of this arrangement?"(18). Regarding the recent educational conference and industry support of CME in general, Dr. Fowler feels comfortable with his answers to these questions.

A similar version of this case study was originally published in ACP Observer in June 1993.

REFERENCES

1. Office of National Cost Estimates. National health expenditures, 1988. Health Care Financing Review. 1990;11:1-54.
2. U.S. Senate, Committee on Labor and Human Resources. Advertising, Marketing and Promotional Practices of the Pharmaceutical Industry Hearing. Dec. 11 and 12, 1990. Washington, DC: U.S. Government Printing Office; 1991.
3. American College of Physicians. Physicians and the pharmaceutical industry. Ann Intern Med. 1990;112:624-6.
4. New York Times, Sunday, 21 Feb., 1993, pp. 1 et seq.
5. Food and Drug Administration. Draft policy statement on industry supported scientific and educational activities [docket no. 92N-0434]. Federal Register, Nov. 27, 1992.
6. Council on Ethical and Judicial Affairs. Gifts to physicians from industry. JAMA. 1991;265:501.
7. Pharmaceutical Manufacturers Association. 1992 Directory of Prescription Drug Indigent Programs (advertisement). American Medical News, August 24-31, 1992; pp. 21-4.
8. U.S. General Accounting Office. Prescription Drugs: Companies Typically Charge More in the United States Than in Canada. Washington, DC: General Accounting Office #GAO/HRD-92-110, September 1992.
9. Office of Technology Assessment. Pharmaceutical R&D: Costs, Risks and Rewards. Washington, DC: U.S. Government Printing Office, 1993.
10. Noble RC. Education or promotion? [Letter]. N Engl J Med. 1992;327:363.
11. Waud DR. Pharmaceutical promotions: a free lunch? N Engl J Med. 1992;327:351-3.
12. Morelli D, Koenigsberg MR. Sample medication dispensing in a residency practice. J Fam Pract. 1992;34:42-8.
13. Safavi KT, Hayward RA. Choosing between apples and apples: physicians' choices of prescription drugs that have similar side effects and efficacies. J Gen Intern Med. 1992;7:32-7.
14. Accreditation Council for Continuing Medical Education. Standards for commercial support of continuing medical education. Lake Bluff, Ill.: ACCME, 1992.

15. Code of Pharmaceutical Marketing Practices. Washington, DC: Pharmaceutical Manufacturers Association, 1990.
16. Drake DC, Uhlman M. How the drug industry woos doctors. Philadelphia Inquirer. 14 December 1992; pp. 1 et seq.
17. Berman JL. Physicians and the pharmaceutical industry [Letter]. Ann Intern Med. 1990;113:900.
18. American College of Physicians. Ethics Manual, 3rd ed. Ann Intern Med. 1992; 117:947-60.

ANNOTATED BIBLIOGRAPHY

Accreditation Council for Continuing Medical Education. Standards for commercial support. Chicago: ACCME; 2004. http://www.accme.org (accessed 22 November 2004).

Offers standards for content, independence, supplementary materials, identification of products, educational materials, management of commercial funds, conflicts of interest, disclosure, and financial support of participants in educational activities.

Coyle SL. Physician-industry relations. Part I: Individual physicians Ann Intern Med. 2002;136:396-402; and Coyle SL. Physician-industry relations. Part 2: Organizational issues. Ann Intern Med. 2002;136:403-6.

The American College of Physicians updated position papers on gifts and hospitality for physicians, drug-industry support of continuing medical education, speaking or writing about a company's product, payment for participation clinic-based research, and the role of medical educators and professional societies in this area.

Council on Ethical and Judicial Affairs. Gifts to physicians from industry. JAMA. 1991;266:265:501.

The American Medical Association's views on the acceptability of gifts to physicians.

Pharmaceutical Research and Manufacturers of America. PhRMA code on interactions with healthcare professionals. Washington, DC: 2004. http://www.phrma.org/publications/policy//2004-01-19.391.pdf (accessed 22 November 2004).

Waud, JR. Pharmaceutical promotions: a free lunch? N Engl J Med. 1992;327:351-3.

Supports professional persuasion rather than regulation or legislation to encourage appropriate physician behavior and finds that no gift is an acceptable gift, which the author views as bribes.

INDEX